Obstructive Sleep Apnea

Obstructive Sleep Apnea

Epidemiology, Pathomechanism and Treatment

Special Issue Editors

Andras Bikov
Silvano Dragonieri

MDPI • Basel • Beijing • Wuhan • Barcelona • Belgrade • Manchester • Tokyo • Cluj • Tianjin

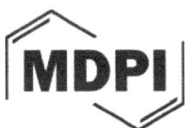

Special Issue Editors

Andras Bikov
University of Manchester
UK

Silvano Dragonieri
University of Bari
Italy

Editorial Office
MDPI
St. Alban-Anlage 66
4052 Basel, Switzerland

This is a reprint of articles from the Special Issue published online in the open access journal *Medicina* (ISSN 1010-660X) (available at: https://www.mdpi.com/journal/medicina/special_issues/Obstructive_Sleep_Apnea).

For citation purposes, cite each article independently as indicated on the article page online and as indicated below:

LastName, A.A.; LastName, B.B.; LastName, C.C. Article Title. *Journal Name* **Year**, *Article Number*, Page Range.

ISBN 978-3-03936-078-9 (Hbk)
ISBN 978-3-03936-079-6 (PDF)

© 2020 by the authors. Articles in this book are Open Access and distributed under the Creative Commons Attribution (CC BY) license, which allows users to download, copy and build upon published articles, as long as the author and publisher are properly credited, which ensures maximum dissemination and a wider impact of our publications.

The book as a whole is distributed by MDPI under the terms and conditions of the Creative Commons license CC BY-NC-ND.

Contents

About the Special Issue Editors vii

Silvano Dragonieri and Andras Bikov
Obstructive Sleep Apnea: A View from the Back Door
Reprinted from: *Medicina* **2020**, *56*, 208, doi:10.3390/medicina56050208 1

**Ioana Mădălina Zota, Cristian Stătescu, Radu Andy Sascău, Mihai Roca,
Radu Sebastian Gavril, Teodor Flaviu Vasilcu, Daniela Boișteanu, Alexandra Maștaleru,
Alexandra Jitaru, Maria Magdalena Leon Constantin and Florin Mitu**
CPAP Effect on Cardiopulmonary Exercise Testing Performance in Patients with Moderate-Severe OSA and Cardiometabolic Comorbidities
Reprinted from: *Medicina* **2020**, *56*, 80, doi:10.3390/medicina56020080 5

**Renata Marietta Bocskei, Martina Meszaros, Adam Domonkos Tarnoki,
David Laszlo Tarnoki, Laszlo Kunos, Zsofia Lazar and Andras Bikov**
Circulating Soluble Urokinase-Type Plasminogen Activator Receptor in Obstructive Sleep Apnoea
Reprinted from: *Medicina* **2020**, *56*, 77, doi:10.3390/medicina56020077 19

Hakan Celikhisar and Gulay Dasdemir Ilkhan
The Association of Obstructive Sleep Apnea Syndrome and Accident Risk in Heavy Equipment Operators
Reprinted from: *Medicina* **2019**, *55*, 599, doi:10.3390/medicina55090599 29

**Carmen Loredana Ardelean, Sorin Pescariu, Daniel Florin Lighezan, Roxana Pleava,
Sorin Ursoniu, Valentin Nadasan and Stefan Mihaicuta**
Particularities of Older Patients with Obstructive Sleep Apnea and Heart Failure with Mid-Range Ejection Fraction
Reprinted from: *Medicina* **2019**, *55*, 449, doi:10.3390/medicina55080449 37

**Prakash Mathiyalagen, Venkatesh Govindasamy, Anandaraj Rajagopal, Kavita Vasudevan,
Kalaipriya Gunasekaran and Dhananjay Yadav**
Magnitude and Determinants of Patients at Risk of Developing Obstructive Sleep Apnea in a Non-Communicable Disease Clinic
Reprinted from: *Medicina* **2019**, *55*, 391, doi:10.3390/medicina55070391 49

Panaiotis Finamore, Simone Scarlata, Vittorio Cardaci and Raffaele Antonelli Incalzi
Exhaled Breath Analysis in Obstructive Sleep Apnea Syndrome: A Review of the Literature
Reprinted from: *Medicina* **2019**, *55*, 538, doi:10.3390/medicina55090538 59

**Alexia Alexandropoulou, Georgios D. Vavougios, Chrissi Hatzoglou,
Konstantinos I. Gourgoulianis and Sotirios G. Zarogiannis**
Risk Assessment for Self Reported Obstructive Sleep Apnea and Excessive Daytime Sleepiness in a Greek Nursing Staff Population
Reprinted from: *Medicina* **2019**, *55*, 468, doi:10.3390/medicina55080468 79

About the Special Issue Editors

Andras Bikov is a post-doc clinical fellow, a specialist in respiratory medicine and an ESRS-certified somnologist with an academic interest in chronic airway diseases and sleep medicine. He graduated as a medical doctor from Semmelweis University, Budapest, Hungary, in 2009, and he completed his PhD training on exhaled breath analysis in 2014 under the supervision of Prof. Ildiko Horvath. As part of his PhD, he received a long-term fellowship from the European Respiratory Society at the National Heart and Lung Institute, Imperial College London, under the supervision of Prof. Peter Barnes. He received his board certificate in respiratory medicine in 2017 and ESRS certification in somnology in 2019. He is currently a consultant in respiratory medicine with a special interest in sleep and ventilation at the Wythenshawe Hospital, Manchester University NHS Foundation Trust, an honorary research physician at the Medicines Evaluation Unit and an honorary clinical fellow at the Division of Infection, Immunity & Respiratory Medicine working in the group led by Professor Jorgen Vestbo. Dr Bikov's research currently focuses on the pathomechanism of COPD using various methods, including the forced oscillation technique, exhaled breath analysis, induced sputum and bronchoalveolar lavage. He has contributed to more than 60 research papers, including the European Respiratory Society technical standard document on exhaled breath analyses. He has an H-index of 16 on Scopus. He is a regular reviewer for many respiratory journals, editor-in-chief for Asthma Research and Practice and an editorial board member for the *Journal of Asthma*. Dr. Bikov is actively involved in the European Respiratory Society, having served as the Early Career Members representative for Assembly 5 (Airway Diseases) between 2013 and 2016.

Silvano Dragonieri is a researcher, assistant professor at the University of Bari, Italy, and a pulmonologist at the University Hospital Policlinico, Bari, Italy. He graduated as a medical doctor from the University of Bari, Italy, in 2003, specialized in Pulmonology at the University of Bari in 2007 and completed his PhD training in 2012 under the supervision of Prof. Peter Sterk at the University of Amsterdam, Netherlands, on exhaled breath analysis by electronic nose. He has contributed to more than 50 research papers. He has an H-index of 16 on Scopus and is a regular reviewer for many respiratory journals. Dr Dragonieri Bikov is an active member of the European Respiratory Society in Assembly 5.2 (Monitoring Airway Diseases).

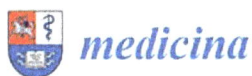

Editorial

Obstructive Sleep Apnea: A View from the Back Door

Silvano Dragonieri [1,*] **and Andras Bikov** [2,3,*]

[1] Department of Respiratory Diseases, University of Bari, 70124 Bari, Italy
[2] North West Lung Centre, Manchester University NHS Foundation Trust, Manchester M239LT, UK
[3] Division of Infection, Immunity and Respiratory Medicine, University of Manchester, Manchester M239LT, UK
* Correspondence: silvano.dragonieri@uniba.it (S.D.); andras.bikov@gmail.com (A.B.)

Received: 22 April 2020; Accepted: 23 April 2020; Published: 25 April 2020

Abstract: Obstructive sleep apnea (OSA) is a common disease that may affect up to 50% of the adult population and whose incidence continues to rise, as well as its health and socio-economic burden. OSA is a well-known risk factor for motor vehicles accidents and decline in work performance and it is frequently accompanied by cardiovascular diseases. The aim of this Special Issue is to focus on the characteristics of OSA in special populations which are less frequently investigated. In this regard, seven groups of experts in the field of sleep medicine gave their contribution in the realization of noteworthy manuscripts which will support all physicians in improving their understanding of OSA with the latest knowledge about its epidemiology, pathophysiology and comorbidities in special populations, which will serve as a basis for future research.

Keywords: obstructive sleep apnea; sleep disordered breathing; cardiovascular comorbidities; biomarkers; inflammation; volatile organic compounds; accident risk; non-communicable diseases; risk assessment

1. Introduction

Obstructive sleep apnea (OSA) is a common disease that may affect up to 50% of the adult population [1]. These percentages are comparable to arterial hypertension [2], and even higher than in diabetes mellitus [3]. Although the exact prevalence in different communities is still unknown, the incidence of OSA continues to rise, as well as its health and socio-economic burden [4]. This Special Issue focuses on the characteristics of OSA in special populations which are less frequently investigated.

OSA is a well-known risk factor for motor vehicles accidents and decline in work performance [5,6]. Alexandropolou et al. concluded that OSA affects around 20% of the Greek nurses and 8% of the nurses have OSA with excessive daytime sleepiness [7]. Celikhisar et al. studied 965 heavy equipment operators in Turkey and found that around 7% of them had OSA [8]. More importantly, the severity of OSA was directly related to the number of work-related accidents [8].

Despite the increasing awareness of OSA and its consequences, most of the patients with OSA remain undiagnosed and untreated [9]. Data on OSA prevalence mainly originate from high-income countries with good healthcare access [4]. In contrast, low- or middle-income countries are less-represented in epidemiological studies. Mathiyalagen et al. screened a population of patients attending non-communicable disease clinics in a rural health training center in South India and reported a 25.8% incidence of OSA [10].

Cardiovascular diseases frequently accompany OSA [11]. Chronic intermittent hypoxia in OSA leads to airway inflammation [12] which can be analyzed in exhaled breath samples [13]. In this issue,

Finamore et al. provide a comprehensive summary on the current knowledge of exhaled breath analysis in OSA [14]. Airway inflammation, together with intermittent hypoxia and surges in the sympathetic activity, induce systemic inflammation [15] which could be a potential link to cardiovascular diseases in OSA. The soluble urokinase type plasminogen activator receptor (suPAR) is a promising biomarker of cardiovascular disease [16]. However, Bocskei et al. reported unaltered suPAR levels in OSA [17]. Despite the relationship between cardiovascular disease and OSA, little is known about the characteristics of obstructive sleep apnea in special subgroups of patients. Ardelean et al. studied 143 patients with heart failure and OSA [18]. They concluded that patients with mid-range ejection fraction (40%–49%) are characterized by a different profile of comorbidities compared to low and preserved ejection fraction subgroups [18]. Finally, in their excellent study, Zota el al. concluded that OSA is related to exercise limitation which is improved after continuous positive airway treatment [19].

Taken together, these studies will support all physicians in improving their understanding of OSA with the latest knowledge about its epidemiology, pathophysiology and comorbidities in special populations, which will serve as a basis for future research.

Acknowledgments: Andras Bikov is supported by the NIHR Manchester BRC.

References

1. Heinzer, R.; Vat, S.; Marques-Vidal, P.; Marti-Soler, H.; Andries, D.; Tobback, N.; Mooser, V.; Preisig, M.; Malhotra, A.; Waeber, G.; et al. Prevalence of sleep-disordered breathing in the general population: The HypnoLaus study. *Lancet Respir. Med.* **2015**, *3*, 310–318.
2. Whelton, P.K.; Carey, R.M.; Aronow, W.S.; Casey, D.E., Jr.; Collins, K.J.; Dennison Himmelfarb, C.; DePalma, S.M.; Gidding, S.; Jamerson, K.A.; Jones, D.W.; et al. 2017 ACC/AHA/AAPA/ABC/ACPM/AGS/APhA/ASH/ASPC/NMA/PCNA Guideline for the Prevention, Detection, Evaluation, and Management of High Blood Pressure in Adults: Executive Summary: A Report of the American College of Cardiology/American Heart Association Task Force on Clinical Practice Guidelines. *Hypertension* **2018**, *71*, 1269–1324.
3. Pinchevsky, Y.; Butkow, N.; Raal, F.J.; Chirwa, T.; Rothberg, A. Demographic and Clinical Factors Associated with Development of Type 2 Diabetes: A Review of the Literature. *Int. J. Gen. Med.* **2020**, *13*, 121–129.
4. Senaratna, C.V.; Perret, J.L.; Lodge, C.J.; Lowe, A.J.; Campbell, B.E.; Matheson, M.C.; Hamilton, G.S.; Dharmage, S.C. Prevalence of obstructive sleep apnea in the general population: A systematic review. *Sleep Med. Rev.* **2017**, *34*, 70–81.
5. Garbarino, S.; Guglielmi, O.; Sanna, A.; Mancardi, G.L.; Magnavita, N. Risk of Occupational Accidents in Workers with Obstructive Sleep Apnea: Systematic Review and Meta-analysis. *Sleep* **2016**, *39*, 1211–1218.
6. Garbarino, S.; Pitidis, A.; Giustini, M.; Taggi, F.; Sanna, A. Motor vehicle accidents and obstructive sleep apnea syndrome: A methodology to calculate the related burden of injuries. *Chronic Respir. Dis.* **2015**, *12*, 320–328.
7. Alexandropoulou, A.; Vavougios, G.D.; Hatzoglou, C.; Gourgoulianis, K.I.; Zarogiannis, S.G. Risk Assessment for Self Reported Obstructive Sleep Apnea and Excessive Daytime Sleepiness in a Greek Nursing Staff Population. *Medicina* **2019**, *55*, 468.
8. Celikhisar, H.; Dasdemir Ilkhan, G. The Association of Obstructive Sleep Apnea Syndrome and Accident Risk in Heavy Equipment Operators. *Medicina* **2019**, *55*, E599.
9. Simpson, L.; Hillman, D.R.; Cooper, M.N.; Ward, K.L.; Hunter, M.; Cullen, S.; James, A.; Palmer, L.J.; Mukherjee, S.; Eastwood, P. High prevalence of undiagnosed obstructive sleep apnoea in the general population and methods for screening for representative controls. *Sleep Breath. Schlaf Atm.* **2013**, *17*, 967–973.
10. Mathiyalagen, P.; Govindasamy, V.; Rajagopal, A.; Vasudevan, K.; Gunasekaran, K.; Yadav, D. Magnitude and Determinants of Patients at Risk of Developing Obstructive Sleep Apnea in a Non-Communicable Disease Clinic. *Medicina* **2019**, *55*, E391.
11. Drager, L.F.; Togeiro, S.M.; Polotsky, V.Y.; Lorenzi-Filho, G. Obstructive sleep apnea: A cardiometabolic risk in obesity and the metabolic syndrome. *J. Am. Coll. Cardiol.* **2013**, *62*, 569–576.

12. Bikov, A.; Hull, J.H.; Kunos, L. Exhaled breath analysis, a simple tool to study the pathophysiology of obstructive sleep apnoea. *Sleep Med. Rev.* **2016**, *27*, 1–8.
13. Dragonieri, S.; Porcelli, F.; Longobardi, F.; Carratu, P.; Aliani, M.; Ventura, V.A.; Tutino, M.; Quaranta, V.N.; Resta, O.; de Gennaro, G. An electronic nose in the discrimination of obese patients with and without obstructive sleep apnoea. *J. Breath Res.* **2015**, *9*, 026005.
14. Finamore, P.; Scarlata, S.; Cardaci, V.; Incalzi, R.A. Exhaled Breath Analysis in Obstructive Sleep Apnea Syndrome: A Review of the Literature. *Medicina* **2019**, *55*, E538.
15. Unnikrishnan, D.; Jun, J.; Polotsky, V. Inflammation in sleep apnea: An update. *Rev. Endocr. Metab. Disord.* **2015**, *16*, 25–34.
16. Eapen, D.J.; Manocha, P.; Ghasemzadeh, N.; Patel, R.S.; Al Kassem, H.; Hammadah, M.; Veledar, E.; Le, N.A.; Pielak, T.; Thorball, C.W.; et al. Soluble urokinase plasminogen activator receptor level is an independent predictor of the presence and severity of coronary artery disease and of future adverse events. *J. Am. Heart Assoc.* **2014**, *3*, e001118.
17. Bocskei, R.M.; Meszaros, M.; Tarnoki, A.D.; Tarnoki, D.L.; Kunos, L.; Lazar, Z.; Bikov, A. Circulating Soluble Urokinase-Type Plasminogen Activator Receptor in Obstructive Sleep Apnoea. *Medicina* **2020**, *56*, E77.
18. Ardelean, C.L.; Pescariu, S.; Lighezan, D.F.; Pleava, R.; Ursoniu, S.; Nadasan, V.; Mihaicuta, S. Particularities of Older Patients with Obstructive Sleep Apnea and Heart Failure with Mid-Range Ejection Fraction. *Medicina* **2019**, *55*, E449.
19. Zota, I.M.; Statescu, C.; Sascau, R.A.; Roca, M.; Gavril, R.S.; Vasilcu, T.F.; Boisteanu, D.; Mastaleru, A.; Jitaru, A.; Leon Constantin, M.M.; et al. CPAP Effect on Cardiopulmonary Exercise Testing Performance in Patients with Moderate-Severe OSA and Cardiometabolic Comorbidities. *Medicina* **2020**, *56*, E80

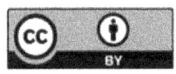

© 2020 by the authors. Licensee MDPI, Basel, Switzerland. This article is an open access article distributed under the terms and conditions of the Creative Commons Attribution (CC BY) license (http://creativecommons.org/licenses/by/4.0/).

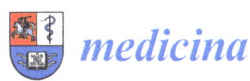

Article

CPAP Effect on Cardiopulmonary Exercise Testing Performance in Patients with Moderate-Severe OSA and Cardiometabolic Comorbidities

Ioana Mădălina Zota [1,†], Cristian Stătescu [1], Radu Andy Sascău [1], Mihai Roca [1,*], Radu Sebastian Gavril [1], Teodor Flaviu Vasilcu [1], Daniela Boișteanu [2], Alexandra Maștaleru [1], Alexandra Jitaru [1], Maria Magdalena Leon Constantin [1] and Florin Mitu [1]

[1] Department of Medical Specialties (I), Faculty of Medicine, Grigore T. Popa—University of Medicine and Pharmacy, 700115 Iași, Romania; madalina.chiorescu@gmail.com (I.M.Z.); cstatescu@gmail.com (C.S.); radu.sascau@gmail.com (R.A.S.); rgavril87@yahoo.com (R.S.G.); teodor.vasilcu@gmail.com (T.F.V.); alexandra.mastaleru@gmail.com (A.M.); alexandrajitaru@gmail.com (A.J.); leon_mariamagdalena@yahoo.com (M.M.L.C.); mitu.florin@yahoo.com (F.M.)
[2] Department of Medical Specialties (III), Faculty of Medicine, Grigore T. Popa—University of Medicine and Pharmacy, 700115 Iași, Romania; boisteanu@yahoo.com
* Correspondence: roca2m@gmail.com
† The study was part of the Ph.D. Thesis of Zota Ioana Mădălina.

Received: 27 January 2020; Accepted: 12 February 2020; Published: 15 February 2020

Abstract: *Background and Objectives:* Obstructive sleep apnea (OSA) is associated with daytime somnolence, cognitive impairment and high cardiovascular morbidity and mortality. Obesity, associated cardiovascular comorbidities, accelerated erythropoiesis and muscular mitochondrial energetic dysfunctions negatively influence exercise tolerance in moderate-severe OSA patients. The cardiopulmonary exercise testing (CPET) offers an integrated assessment of the individual's aerobic capacity and helps distinguish the main causes of exercise limitation. The purpose of this study is to evaluate the aerobic capacity of OSA patients, before and after short-term continuous positive airway pressure (CPAP). *Materials and Methods:* Our prospective study included 64 patients with newly diagnosed moderate-severe OSA (apnea hypopnea index (AHI) 39.96 ± 19.04 events/h) who underwent CPET before and after CPAP. Thirteen patients were unable to tolerate CPAP or were lost during follow-up. Results: 49.29% of our patients exhibited a moderate or severe decrease in functional capacity (Weber C or D). CPET performance was influenced by gender but not by apnea severity. Eight weeks of CPAP induced significant improvements in maximal exercise load (Δ = 14.23 W, p = 0.0004), maximum oxygen uptake (Δ = 203.87 mL/min, p = 0.004), anaerobic threshold (Δ = 316.4 mL/min, p = 0.001), minute ventilation (Δ = 5.1 L/min, p = 0.01) and peak oxygen pulse (Δ = 2.46, p = 0.007) as well as a decrease in basal metabolic rate (BMR) (Δ = −8.3 kCal/24 h, p = 0.04) and average Epworth score (Δ = −4.58 points, p < 0.000001). *Conclusions:* Patients with moderate-severe OSA have mediocre functional capacity. Apnea severity (AHI) was correlated with basal metabolic rate, resting heart rate and percent predicted maximum effort but not with anaerobic threshold or maximum oxygen uptake. Although CPET performance was similar in the two apnea severity subgroups, short-term CPAP therapy significantly improved most CPET parameters, suggesting that OSA per se has a negative influence on effort capacity.

Keywords: obstructive sleep apnea; continuous positive airway treatment; cardiopulmonary exercise testing; functional capacity; cardiovascular rehabilitation

1. Introduction

Repetitive nocturnal upper airway collapse, with subsequent hypoxic episodes and microawakenings, is the hallmark of obstructive sleep apnea (OSA) [1]. While chronic sleep fragmentation leads to excessive daytime somnolence and cognitive impairment [2], hypoxia is associated with autonomic and hormonal imbalance, endothelial dysfunction and oxidative stress [3], explaining the high cardiovascular morbidity and mortality described among OSA patients [1,3].

In-hospital polysomnography is the diagnostic standard for OSA, with cardio-respiratory polygraphy considered an acceptable alternative [4–6]. According to the apnea–hypopnea index (AHI), defined as the number of apneic or hypopneic episodes per hour of sleep, OSA is classified as mild, moderate or severe [7]. Daytime sleepiness is the main symptom in OSA, a subjective parameter that can be objectively assessed using the Epworth questionnaire.

Treatment is recommended in all cases of moderate-severe OSA (AHI ≥ 15 events/h), as well as in patients with mild OSA who associate symptoms or cerebrovascular comorbidities [8]. Current therapy options include continuous positive airway pressure (CPAP), mandibular advancement devices, maxillo-facial surgery and nocturnal hypoglossal nerve stimulation [9,10]. Although CPAP remains the gold-standard treatment option for moderate-severe OSA, its use is limited by poor treatment adherence, especially among children.

Obesity and weight-related lung-function abnormalities (decreased functional residual capacity and expiratory reserve volume, impaired respiratory system compliance) are highly prevalent among OSA patients [10]. Associated cardiovascular comorbidities (hypertension, heart failure, pulmonary hypertension), hypoxia-induced erythropoiesis [11] with subsequent hematological alterations and muscular mitochondrial dysfunctions also contribute to a decreased exercise tolerance [10,12]. The cardiopulmonary exercise testing (CPET) provides an integrative assessment of the cardiopulmonary, muscular, neuropsychological and hematopoietic systems, which directly impact the individual's functional capacity [13]. CPET is a valuable cardiovascular instrument for risk stratification and prognosis assessment, helping to establish a personalized exercise training program for OSA patients. Current literature [14] offers conflicting results regarding CPET results in OSA patients and the role of CPAP in improving exercise performance. As such, the purpose of this study is to evaluate the impact of short-term (8 weeks) CPAP therapy on exercise capacity of patients with moderate-severe OSA and cardiometabolic comorbidities.

2. Materials and Methods

We performed a prospective study that included newly diagnosed patients with moderate-severe OSA (prior to the initiation of CPAP therapy), admitted in our local cardiovascular rehabilitation clinic between October 2017 and December 2018. OSA diagnosis was made by ambulatory or in-hospital six-channel cardio-respiratory polygraphy, using either a Philips Respironics Alice Night One or a DeVilbiss Porti 7 device. The recordings were manually scored by a trained physician, according to the American Academy of Sleep Medicine (AASM) standards. Patients with an apnea–hypopnea index (AHI) of 15–30 and >30 were considered to have moderate and severe OSA, respectively. A Philips Respironics DreamStation Auto CPAP or a Resmed Airsense 10 Autoset were used for CPAP effective pressure autotitration in the sleep laboratory.

All patients signed a written informed consent for inclusion. The study was conducted in accordance with the Declaration of Helsinki, and the protocol was approved by the Ethics Committee of the "Grigore T. Popa" University of Medicine and Pharmacy in Iași (ethical approval code 1183). All subjects underwent physical examination, lipid profile, cardiopulmonary exercise testing and were asked to complete the Epworth questionnaire, before and after 2 months of CPAP therapy. Obesity was defined as a body mass index (BMI ≥ 30 kg/m^2). High blood pressure (HBP) was defined as current BP lowering treatment, prior diagnosis of HBP or resting BP values greater than 140 and 90 mmHg for systolic and diastolic BP, respectively. Dyslipidemia was defined as total cholesterol ≥ 200 mg/dL and/or triglycerides ≥ 150 mg/dL. Ischemic heart disease was defined as history of myocardial infarction or prior angiographically documented significant coronary artery stenosis. According to the results of the Epworth questionnaire, daytime sleepiness was categorized as normal, mild, moderate and severe (0–10 points, 11–12 points, 13–15 points and 16–24 points, respectively). Functional capacity was assessed according to peak oxygen uptake (VO2), using the Weber classification, as follows: Weber A (little or no impairment): >20 mL/kg/min, Weber B (mild to moderate impairment): 16–20 mL/kg/min, Weber C (moderate to severe impairment): 10–16 mL/kg/min and Weber D (severe impairment) < 10 mL/kg/min.

CPET was performed under the direction of a certified pulmonologist on the Piston PRE-201 ergospirometer. This started with a 2 min resting period followed by 1 min warm up pedaling against no resistance and an incremental test protocol of 10 W/min. The CPET was performed under continuous heart rate (HR), ECG (electrocardiographic) and pulse oximetry (SpO2) monitoring. BP was recorded every 2 min. Indications for exercise termination included extreme fatigue, myocardial ischemia, complex ventricular premature beats, grade 2 or grade 3 atrio-ventricular block, a sudden drop in BP levels by more than 20 mmHg, increased BP (systolic blood pressure (SBP) > 220 mmHg, diastolic blood pressure (DBP) > 120 mmHg), SpO2 < 80%, confusion, dizziness and sudden pallor.

Statistical analysis was performed in SPSS v. 20.0, using chi-square and student's t-test for comparisons between groups. A potential relationship between variables was evaluated using Pearson's correlation coefficient. The ANCOVA test was used for BMI-adjusted comparison of CPET performance before and after CPAP use. Descriptive data were expressed as means ± SD (standard deviation) or percentages, as appropriate. A p value < 0.05 was considered statistically significant.

3. Results

Our initial study group included 64 patients aged 36–79 years old (57.53 ± 8.74 years old), mean BMI 34.04 ± 5.30 kg/m^2, with newly diagnosed OSA (AHI 39.96 ± 19.04 events/h, desaturation index 38.67 ± 19.67 events/h, average nocturnal SpO2 91.63% ± 3.64%, CPAP pressure 11.27 ± 2.43 cmH20). Almost two-thirds of our study group presented severe OSA (59.37%) (Figure 1). Male sex was predominant in our study group, with a M/F ratio of 2.55 (Figure 2). Cardiometabolic comorbidities (particularly hypertension) were highly prevalent among our patients (Figure 3).

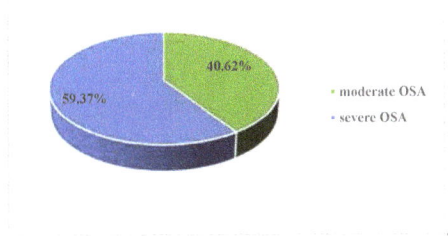

Figure 1. Prevalence of moderate and severe obstructive sleep apnea (OSA) in our study group.

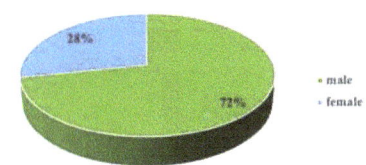

Figure 2. Gender distribution in our study group.

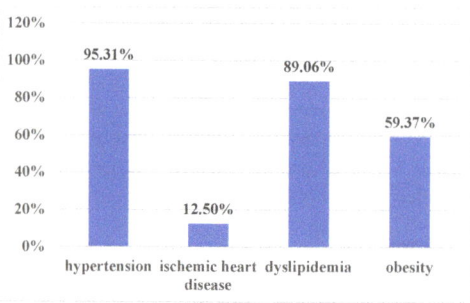

Figure 3. Prevalence of cardio-metabolic comorbidities in our study group.

Of our patients, 49.21% exhibited a moderate or severe decrease in functional capacity, according to the Weber classification (Weber C or D) (Figure 4). Only one in five patients with moderate-severe OSA had a normal functional capacity (Weber A). We found no significant differences regarding average AHI values between the four functional capacity subgroups (Weber A to D) ($p > 0{,}05$).

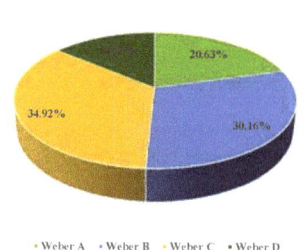

Figure 4. Functional capacity in our study group according to the Weber classification.

Apart from maximal instantaneous forced expiratory flow (MEF)25% that was higher in the severe OSA subgroup, we did not find any statistically significant differences regarding spirometry results between patients with moderate and severe OSA (Table 1).

Table 1. Spirometry results in patients with moderate-severe OSA.

	Moderate-Severe OSA		Moderate OSA		Severe OSA		p
	Average	SD	Average	SD	Average	SD	
FVC (L)	3.76	0.92	3.84	0.85	3.71	0.97	0.46
FVC% (%)	94.89	19.03	94.00	18.47	95.45	19.67	0.79
FEV1.0 (L)	3.05	0.68	3.12	0.66	3.00	0.69	0.54
FEV 1.0% (%)	91.61	19.96	88.00	19.39	93.90	20.30	0.31
FEV1.0/FVC	77.24	2.12	77.54	1.86	77.06	2.28	0.44
FEV1.0/FVC%	101.20	10.82	97.67	11.79	103.32	9.80	0.07
PEF (L/sec)	7.64	1.37	7.73	1.31	7.59	1.42	0.72
PEF% (%)	77.00	19.63	75.22	18.92	78.07	20.28	0.63
MEF 25 (L/sec)	1.59	0.39	1.65	0.37	1.55	0.41	0.43
MEF 25% (%)	69.90	23.39	61.17	24.04	75.33	21.64	0.04
MEF 50 (L/sec)	4.22	0.61	4.28	0.58	4.17	0.63	0.56
MEF 50% (%)	75.93	25.80	68.11	27.96	80.78	23.56	0.10
MEF 75 (L/sec)	6.74	1.16	6.80	1.12	6.69	1.20	0.75
MEF 75% (%)	76.44	20.75	72.89	21.67	78.65	20.22	0.36

FVC—forced vital capacity; FVC%—percent predicted forced vital capacity; FEV1—forced expiratory volume in one second; FEV1%—percent predicted forced expiratory volume in one second; PEF—peak expiratory flow; PEF%—percent predicted peak expiratory flow; MEF—maximal instantaneous forced expiratory flow; MEF%—percent predicted maximal instantaneous forced expiratory flow.

CPET performance was influenced by gender but not by apnea severity (Tables 2 and 3).

Table 2. Gender influence on cardiopulmonary exercise testing (CPET) parameters among patients with moderate-severe OSA.

	Male		Female		p
	Average	SD	Average	SD	
BMR (kCal/24 h)	1860.18	264.14	1494.06	187.26	<0.0000001
Maximal load (W)	114.85	33.54	80.78	23.41	0.0001
% predicted maximal load	56.74	16.04	70.07	15.49	0.004
VO2 max	1553.20	504.55	1301.67	352.11	0.07
% predicted VO2 max	61.59	21.73	81.83	15.56	0.0005
AT	1202.82	397.46	1083.07	288.10	0.33
Weight-indexed AT	11.82	3.79	11.83	3.15	0.99
VCO2 max	1434.52	460.30	1392.83	330.89	0.75
VE max (L/min)	48.64	12.88	40.29	8.79	0.02
Resting HR	79.20	12.27	83.80	15.85	0.21
Peak HR	117.02	19.34	123.73	18.52	0.25
% predicted peak HR	71.48	11.62	77.80	11.29	0.07
Peak O2 pulse	14.46	5.46	12.37	5.40	0.20
Weight-indexed O2 pulse	0.14	0.06	0.14	0.07	0.97
Baseline SBP	124.72	16.05	127.87	16.12	0.51
Baseline DBP	78.46	9.83	79.27	13.29	0.78
Peak SBP	183.16	28.01	185.33	18.85	0.80
Peak DBP	98.64	17.61	102.53	9.52	0.46

CPET—cardiopulmonary stress test; OSA—obstructive sleep apnea; BMR—basal metabolic rate; VO2—peak oxygen uptake; AT—anaerobic threshold; VCO2—peak CO2 output; VE—minute ventilation; HR—heart rate; SBP—systolic blood pressure; DBP—diastolic blood pressure.

Table 3. Differences regarding CPET parameters between moderate and severe OSA subgroups.

	Moderate-Severe OSA		Moderate OSA		Severe OSA		p
	Average	SD	Average	SD	Average	SD	
BMR (kCal/24 h)	1755.57	264.14	1726.27	276.57	1776.16	256.87	0.46
Maximal load (W)	105.27	33.54	111.08	34.20	101.29	32.94	0.25
% predicted maximal load	60.02	16.04	61.84	13.81	58.75	17.50	0.46
VO2 max	1482.45	504.55	1464.31	473.61	1494.87	530.57	0.81
% predicted VO2 max	67.28	21.73	67.27	21.98	67.29	21.86	0.99
AT	1168.92	397.46	1109.32	367.95	1211.23	417.85	0.36
Weight-indexed AT	11.83	3.79	11.59	4.24	12.00	3.49	0.70
VCO2 max	1422.80	460.30	1421.54	476.78	1423.66	455.16	0.98
VE max (L/min)	46.58	12.88	47.12	9.21	46.21	15.03	0.78
%VE	43.05	12.51	41.89	15.86	44.05	10.40	0.57
Resting HR	80.33	12.27	77.88	11.59	82.03	12.59	0.19
Peak HR	118.67	19.34	121.84	18.81	116.47	19.66	0.29
% predicted maximum HR	73.03	11.62	74.68	11.70	71.89	11.59	0.36
Peak O2 pulse	13.95	5.46	14.00	5.34	13.91	5.62	0.95
Weight-indexed O2 pulse	0.14	0.06	0.15	0.06	0.14	0.06	0.42
Baseline SBP	125.49	16.05	120.04	11.64	129.28	17.69	0.02
Baseline DBP	78.66	9.83	76.88	7.32	79.89	11.18	0.24
Peak SBP	183.70	28.01	175.50	26.32	189.17	28.12	0.06
Peak DBP	99.62	17.61	97.79	13.01	100.83	20.20	0.51

CPET—cardiopulmonary stress test; OSA—obstructive sleep apnea; BMR—basal metabolic rate; VO2—peak oxygen uptake; AT—anaerobic threshold; VCO2—peak CO2 output; VE—minute ventilation; HR—heart rate; SBP—systolic blood pressure; DBP—diastolic blood pressure.

Except for baseline SBP, CPET parameters did not significantly differ between the two apnea severity subgroups (Table 2). Basal metabolic rate (BMR) and minute ventilation (VE) max were significantly higher among males (Δ = 366 kCal/24 h and Δ = 8.35 L/min, respectively). Although males achieved a higher average peak workload (Δ = 34.07 W), % predicted workload and % predicted VO2 max were significantly higher in the female subgroup (Δ = 13.33% and Δ = 20.24%, respectively).

Apnea severity was significantly correlated with resting HR ($r = -0.30$, $p = 0,01$) (Figure 5), % predicted workload ($r = -0.30$, $p = 0.01$) (Figure 6) and BMR ($r = 0.33$, $p = 0.008$) (Figure 7) (Table 4).

We did not find any statistically significant correlations between AHI and the analyzed spirometry parameters ($p > 0.05$).

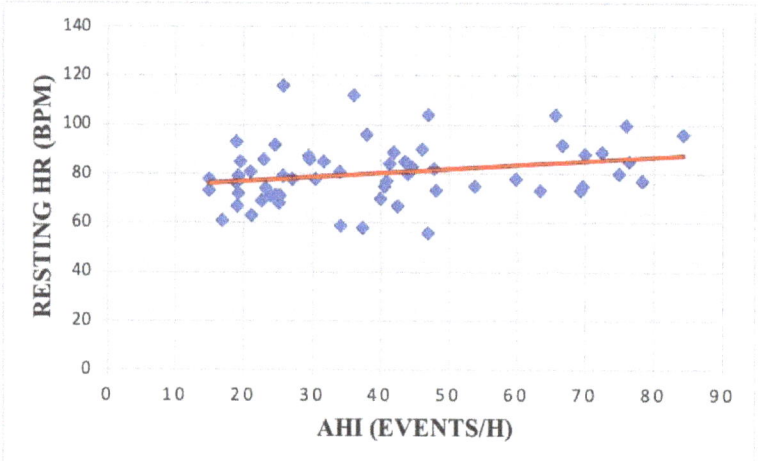

Figure 5. Correlation between apnea severity and resting heart rate among patients with moderate-severe OSA ($r = 0.25$, $p = 0.04$). HR—heart rate; AHI—apnea hypopnea index; OSA—obstructive sleep apnea.

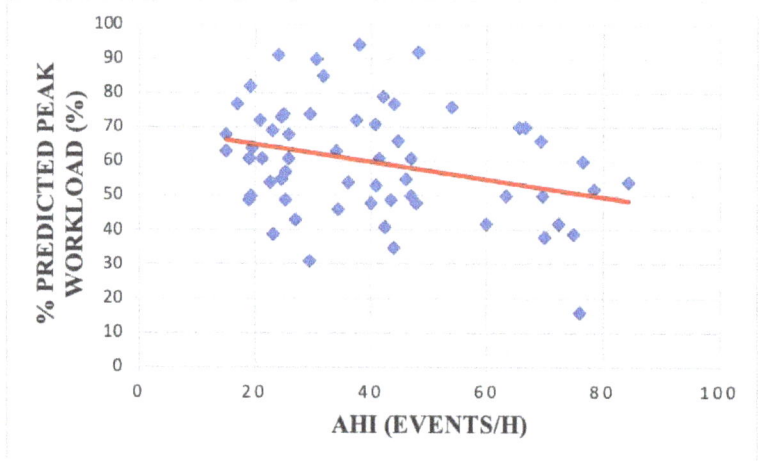

Figure 6. Correlation between apnea severity and % predicted peak workload among patients with moderate-severe OSA ($r = -0.30$, $p = 0.01$). AHI—apnea hypopnea index; OSA—obstructive sleep apnea.

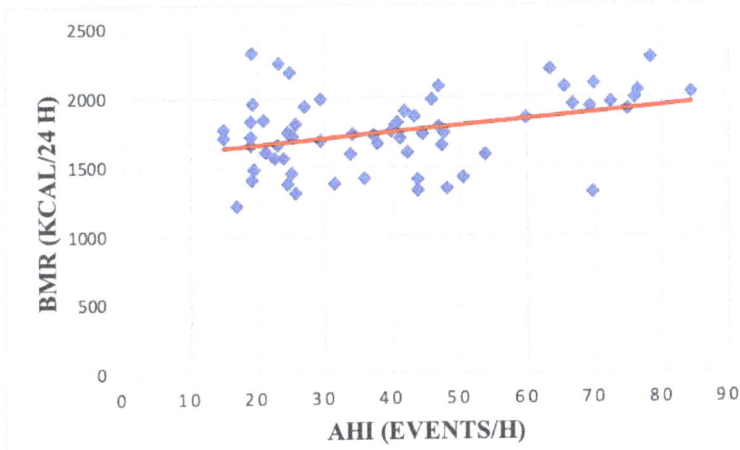

Figure 7. Correlation between apnea severity and BMR among patients with moderate-severe OSA ($r = 0.33$, $p = 0.008$). BMR—basal metabolic rate; AHI—apnea hypopnea index; OSA—obstructive sleep apnea.

Table 4. Correlations between AHI and CPET results among patients with moderate-severe OSA.

	r	p		r	p
BMR (kCal/24 h)	0.33	0.008	VCO2 max	0.10	0.42
Maximal load (W)	−0.07	0.55	VE max (L/min)	0.05	0.72
% predicted maximal load	−0.30	0.01	Resting HR	0.25	0.04
VO2 max	0.02	0.88	Peak HR	−0.12	0.33
% predicted VO2 max	−0.20	0.10	% predicted peak HR	−0.21	0.09
AT	0.15	0.28	Peak O2 pulse	−0.05	0.67
Weight-indexed AT	−0.02	0.85	Weight-indexed O2 pulse	−0.19	0.13

AHI—apnea hypopnea index; CPET—cardiopulmonary stress test; OSA—obstructive sleep apnea; BMR—basal metabolic rate; VO2—peak oxygen uptake; AT—anaerobic threshold; VCO2—peak CO2 output; VE—minute ventilation; HR—heart rate.

All subjects started appropriate continuous positive airway pressure therapy. Thirteen patients were unable to tolerate CPAP or were lost during follow-up. Fifty-one patients successfully completed the CPET and the Epworth questionnaires before and after 2 months of CPAP.

The average Epworth score in our study group was 8.11 ± 5.23 points. Average CPAP use was 241.67 (±128.38) minutes/night. Only 51.16% of our patients used the device as recommended—at least 4 h/night. CPAP use did not significantly impact basal blood pressure values (SBP Δ = −4.58 mmHg, $p = 0.13$; DBP Δ = −1.52 mmHg, $p = 0.35$) and was not associated with statistically significant weight loss (Δ = −1.01 kg, $p = 0.57$).

After 2 months of CPAP our study group exhibited significant improvements in maximal exercise load (Δ = 14.23 W, $p = 0.0004$), VO2 max (Δ = 203.87 mL/min, $p = 0.004$), anaerobic threshold (AT) (Δ = 316.4 mL/min, $p = 0.001$) and VE max (Δ = 5.1 L/min, $p = 0.01$) (Table 5, Figures 8 and 9). Maximal exercise load and VO2 max improvement remained significant after adjustment for BMI (Table 5. $p = 0.04$ and $p = 0.02$, respectively). We also observed an increase in peak oxygen pulse (Δ = 2.46, $p = 0.007$) and VCO2 max (Δ = 232.14 mL/min, $p = 0.0006$), which remained significant after adjusting for BMI (Table 5, Figures 8 and 9, $p = 0.02$ and $p = 0.01$, respectively). The Epworth score in our study group decreased by 4.58 points ($p < 0.000001$).

Table 5. CPAP impact on CPET parameters in moderate-severe OSA patients.

	Baseline		After CPAP		$p\,*$	$p\,**$
	Average	SD	Average	SD		
BMR (kCal/24 h)	1771.50	281.49	1763.12	273.79	0.04	0.78
Maximal load (W)	103.16	34.21	117.39	36.17	0.0004	0.04
% predicted maximal load	59.83	16.48	68.69	14.35	0.0001	0.01
VO2 max	1458.27	435.29	1662.14	454.50	0.004	0.02
% predicted VO2 max	64.54	17.49	76.82	18.47	0.000005	0.001
AT	1134.30	419.42	1450.70	450.54	0.001	0.08
Weight-indexed AT	11.41	4.07	14.62	4.66	0.001	0.07
VCO2 max	1464.34	383.13	1696.48	465.62	0.0006	0.01
VE max (L/min)	46.46	13.57	51.56	14.23	0.016	0.09
%VE	43.07	12.69	47.52	11.48	0.04	0.04
Resting HR	80.37	13.15	76.19	14.46	0.05	-
Peak HR	118.22	20.06	121.67	23.94	0.28	-
% predicted maximum HR	72.59	11.84	73.84	11.96	0.42	-
Peak O2 pulse	13.59	4.14	16.05	5.83	0.007	0.02
Weight-indexed O2 pulse	0.14	0.05	0.16	0.06	0.01	0.26
Baseline SBP	126.77	17.63	122.19	15.93	0.13	-
Baseline DBP	78.94	10.29	77.42	8.77	0.35	-
Peak SBP	184.62	29.35	185.35	23.27	0.85	-
Peak DBP	101.52	13.74	98.33	10.40	0.11	-

CPAP—continuous positive airway pressure; CPET—cardiopulmonary stress test; OSA—obstructive sleep apnea; BMR—basal metabolic rate; VO2—peak oxygen uptake; AT—anaerobic threshold; VCO2—peak CO2 output; VE—minute ventilation; HR—heart rate; SBP—systolic blood pressure; DBP—diastolic blood pressure; $p\,*$—statistical significance for non-adjusted student's t-test; $p\,**$—statistical significance for BMI-adjusted results of ANCOVA test.

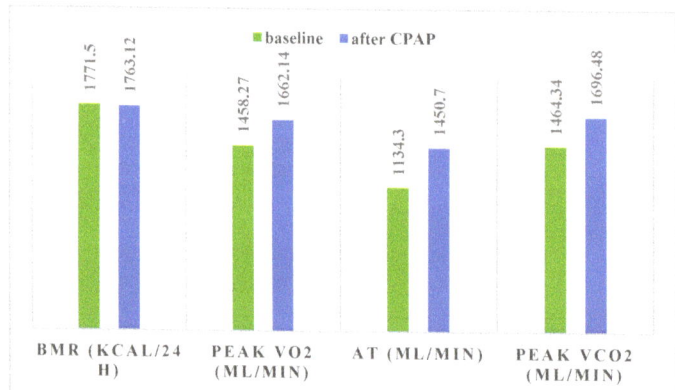

Figure 8. CPAP induced changes in BMR (Δ = −8.38 kCal/24 h, p = 0.04), peak VO2 (Δ = 203.87 mL/min, p = 0.004), AT (Δ = 316.4 mL/min, p = 0.001) and peak VCO2 max (Δ = 232.14 mL/min, p = 0.0006). BMR—basal metabolic rate; peak VO2—peak oxygen uptake; AT—anaerobic threshold; peak VCO2—peak CO2 output.

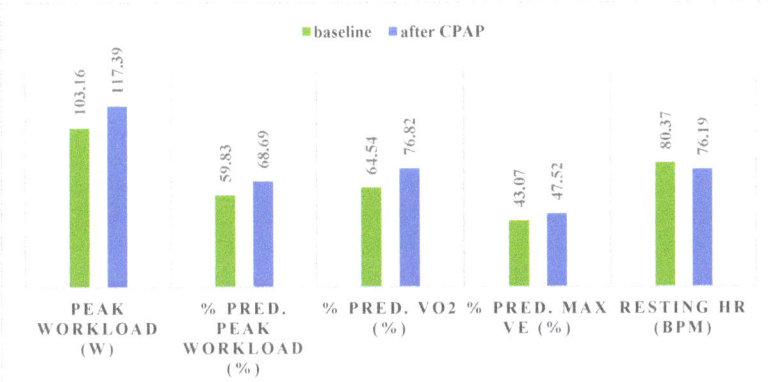

Figure 9. CPAP induced changes in peak workload (Δ = 14.23 W, p = 0.0004), % predicted peak workload (Δ = 8.86 %, p = 0.0001), % predicted peak VO2 (Δ = 12.28 %, p = 0.000005), % predicted VE max (Δ = 4.45 %, p = 0.01) and resting HR (Δ = −4.18 bpm, p = 0.05), in moderate-severe OSA patients. CPAP—continuous positive airway pressure; OSA—obstructive sleep apnea; VO2—peak oxygen uptake; VE—minute ventilation; HR—heart rate.

4. Discussion

Our study included 64 patients aged 57.53 ± 8.74 years old with newly diagnosed moderate-severe OSA. This value is slightly higher than other reports concerning average OSA age at diagnosis (40–50 years old) [15]. Female sex hormones increase genioglossus contractility and prevent upper airway collapsibility during sleep [16,17]. Furthermore, the distinctive distribution of adipose tissue among the two genders (with central obesity being more strongly associated with OSA) [18], as well as the higher pharyngeal resistance in men [19], explain why OSA is more prevalent among male patients. Despite the evident predominance of the male sex in our study group, our male/female ratio is slightly lower than in previous studies (2.55:1 vs. 3:1–5:1) [20].

Similar to other literature reports [21], the main reason for premature test halt was dyspnea accompanied by muscular exhaustion. Extreme fatigue in OSA patients can be explained by the presence of energetic mitochondrial dysfunctions especially in muscle cells [12]. An exaggerated SBP response (SBP > 250 mmHg) was the second reason for premature test halt. None of our patients presented arrhythmic events, confusion or a decrease in BP values during exercise.

Our moderate-severe OSA patients presented baseline mediocre CPET performance. Only 20.63% of our subjects had a baseline normal functional capacity according to the Weber classification, and most cases (34.92%) were classified as moderately impaired. In comparison, Przybyłowski et al. [22] reported an overall better CPET performance in 111 obese OSA patients (% predicted peak VO2 85.3 ± 17.8, peak VCO2 2800 ± 900 mL/min, VE max 91.2 ± 24.7, % predicted maximum HR 92.5 ± 10.3), despite a minimal difference in OSA severity between the two groups (average AHI 47.2 ± 23.1 vs. 39.96 ± 19.04 events/h). However, Przybyłowski's study group included an unusually low percentage of hypertensives (29% vs. 95.31% in our study group), signaling that HBP could be an important confounding factor when analyzing CPET performance.

Previous reports regarding the impact of OSAS on cardiopulmonary exercise testing performance have conflicting results and included a limited number of patients [10,12,23–25]. Most studies that associated OSAS with an impaired exercise capacity (decreased exercise duration, workload, VO2, oxygen pulse, AT and/or VE max) were conducted on obese or overweight subjects [10,12,25]. Therefore, these reports could be biased by the known negative impact of obesity on exercise capacity, as shown by Rizzi et al. [26].

Consistent with this theory, another report [27] found that CPET performance is similar among normoponderal OSAS patients and controls, although it is worth mentioning that the analyzed group had a relatively low average AHI (15.4 ± 9.2) and included an unusually large proportion of females (63%).

Powell et al. [28] studied exercise performance among military personnel with and without moderate-severe OSAS. The lack of significant differences among the two subgroups could be explained by the low average age in the OSAS and control groups (40.7 and 39.4, respectively) but also by the higher grade of habitual physical activity (characteristic for this population subset) [29].

However, a recent meta-analysis [29] has shown that VO2 max is significantly lower in OSA subjects compared to controls (Δ = 2.7 mL/kg/min), the difference being of greater clinical impact among non-obese patients (Δ = 4.1 mL/kg/min).

Rizzi et al. [26] reported that male sex associated with diabetes negatively impacts VO2 max. Consistent with their results, our female subgroup obtained significantly higher percent predicted workload and percent-predicted maximum HR, suggesting a higher effort capacity.

Apnea severity was previously correlated with several CPET parameters including VO2 max [25], percent predicted peak VO2 [30] and BP rise during exercise [22]. However, our analysis only found a significant association between AHI resting HR, BMR and percent predicted workload. The high prevalence of cardio-metabolic comorbidities in our study group (especially obesity and hypertension) could explain the lack of statistically significant correlations between AHI and other CPET variables.

Previous studies [24,25,29] reported that OSAS patients have higher DBP values and decreased HR recovery compared to controls. When analyzing the two apnea severity subgroups, we observed significantly higher baseline and AT-SBP values (but no significant differences regarding HR response during exercise) in the severe OSA subgroup.

Literature reports regarding the impact of CPAP on VO2 max in OSAS patients have yielded inconsistent results. Different CPAP therapy lengths (1 week–8 months) were associated with significant VO2 max improvements [29,31–33]. However, in another study [34], VO2 max displayed a mild negative trend (22.52 ± 6.62 mL/min/kg to 21.32 ± 5.26 mL/min/kg; p = 0.111) in CPAP compliant patients and a borderline statistically significant decline in patients with suboptimal CPAP use (21.31 ± 5.66 mL/min/kg to 19.92 ± 5.40 mL/min/kg, p = 0.05).

Despite a mediocre CPAP adherence (241.67 min/night), our patients exhibited a significant improvement in percent predicted maximum workload, percent predicted VO2 max, AT and oxygen pulse. Improvements regarding maximal load, VO2 max, VCO2 max, %VE and peak O2 pulse remained significant even after adjusting for BMI. We observed no statistically significant gender-related differences regarding these changes. Quadri et al. [33] also studied the effect of 2 months of CPAP in a smaller group of moderate-severe OSAS patients and reported similar improvements in percent predicted maximum workload (9 vs. 8.86 W%) and percent predicted VO2 peak (9.7% vs. 12.28%) but a less marked increase regarding AT (99 vs. 316.4 mL/min). On the other hand, Tapan et al. [21] analyzed the benefit of 8 weeks of CPAP in patients with severe OSA and observed a greater improvement in maximum workload and VE (16.9 W and 10.3 L/min respectively) but a less important increase in percentage-predicted peak VO2 (7.6% vs. 12.28%).

Previous research [35] reported diurnal variations in spirometric indices in OSA patients (especially among males). The same study [35] observed significant associations between AHI, evening forced expiratory volume in one second (FEV1) and forced vital capacity (FVC) and demonstrated the important influence of BMI, hypertension, dyslipidemia and several cardiovascular drugs on the relationship between lung function and apnea severity. The fact that most of our patients presented cardio-metabolic comorbidities, and were under treatment with a statin, beta blocker or a renin-angiotensin-aldosterone axis inhibitor [35], could explain the lack of association between AHI and the analyzed spirometry parameters (p > 0.05).

The main limitations of our study are the lack of a control group and the high prevalence of cardio-metabolic comorbidities among our patients. Although obesity and hypertension are important confounders regarding the decrease in CPET performance described in OSAS patients, the presence of these comorbidities reflects the typical, everyday OSAS patient and, in our opinion, should not be excluded from analysis. Although baseline CPET results did not significantly differ between the two apnea severity subgroups, the fact that our 2 months of CPAP improved most CPET parameters in the absence of statistically significant weight loss ($\Delta = -1.01$ kg, $p = 0.57$) or basal BP changes (SBP $\Delta = -4.58$ mmHg $p = 0.13$; DBP $\Delta = -1.52$ mmHg $p = 0.35$) suggests that OSAS per se impacts exercise capacity.

5. Conclusions

Moderate-severe OSA patients have a mediocre baseline CPET performance. AHI was correlated with some CPET parameters (BMR, % predicted effort, resting HR) but not with VO2 or AT. Two months of CPAP improved most CPET parameters (in the absence of statistically significant weight loss or basal BP changes) suggesting that OSAS per se negatively impacts effort capacity.

Author Contributions: All authors have equally contributed to this work. All authors have read and agreed to the published version of the manuscript.

Funding: This research received no external funding.

Conflicts of Interest: The authors declare no conflict of interest.

References

1. Spicuzza, L.; Caruso, D.; Di Maria, G. Obstructive sleep apnoea syndrome and its management. *Ther. Adv. Chronic Dis.* **2015**, *6*, 273–285. [CrossRef] [PubMed]
2. Gagnon, K.; Baril, A.A.; Gagnon, J.F.; Fortin, M.; Décary, A.; Lafond, C.; Desautels, A.; Montplaisir, J.; Gosselin, N. Cognitive impairment in obstructive sleep apnea. *Pathol. Biol. (Paris)* **2014**, *62*, 233–240. [CrossRef] [PubMed]
3. Drager, L.F.; McEvoy, R.D.; Barbe, F.; Lorenzi-Filho, G.; Redline, S.; INCOSACT Initiative (International Collaboration of Sleep Apnea Cardiovascular Trialists). Sleep Apnea and Cardiovascular Disease: Lessons From Recent Trials and Need for Team Science. *Circulation* **2017**, *136*, 1840–1850. [CrossRef] [PubMed]
4. Lévy, P.; Kohler, M.; McNicholas, W.T.; Barbé, F.; McEvoy, R.D.; Somers, V.K.; Lavie, L.; Pépin, J.-L. Obstructive sleep apnoea syndrome. *Nat. Rev. Dis. Primer.* **2015**, *1*, 15015. [CrossRef]
5. Sateia, M.J. International classification of sleep disorders-third edition: Highlights and modifications. *Chest* **2014**, *146*, 1387–1394. [CrossRef]
6. La Rovere, M.T.; Fanfulla, F.; Febo, O. Obstructive sleep apnea: One more target in cardiac rehabilitation. *Monaldi. Arch. Chest Dis.* **2015**, *82*, 160–164. [CrossRef]
7. Berry, R.B.; Budhiraja, R.; Gottlieb, D.J.; Gozal, D.; Iber, C.; Kapur, V.K.; Marcus, C.L.; Mehra, R.; Parthasarathy, S.; Quan, S.F.; et al. Rules for Scoring Respiratory Events in Sleep: Update of the 2007 AASM Manual for the Scoring of Sleep and Associated Events. *J. Clin. Sleep Med.* **2012**, *8*, 597–619. [CrossRef]
8. Veasey, S.C.; Rosen, I.M. Obstructive Sleep Apnea in Adults. *N. Engl. J. Med.* **2019**, *380*, 1442–1449. [CrossRef]
9. Woodson, B.T.; Strohl, K.P.; Soose, R.J.; Gillespie, M.B.; Maurer, J.T.; de Vries, N.; Padhya, T.A.; Badr, M.S.; Lin, H.-S.; Vanderveken, O.M.; et al. Upper Airway Stimulation for Obstructive Sleep Apnea: 5-Year Outcomes. *Otolaryngol.-Head Neck Surg. Off. J. Am. Acad. Otolaryngol.-Head Neck Surg.* **2018**, *159*, 194–202. [CrossRef]
10. Lin, C.-C.; Hsieh, W.-Y.; Chou, C.-S.; Liaw, S.-F. Cardiopulmonary exercise testing in obstructive sleep apnea syndrome. *Respir. Physiol. Neurobiol.* **2006**, *150*, 27–34. [CrossRef]
11. Khan, A.M.; Ashizawa, S.; Hlebowicz, V.; Appel, D.W. Anemia of aging and obstructive sleep apnea. *Sleep Breath.* **2011**, *15*, 29–34. [CrossRef]
12. Stavrou, V.; Bardaka, F.; Karetsi, E.; Daniil, Z.; Gourgoulianis, K.I. Brief Review: Ergospirometry in Patients with Obstructive Sleep Apnea Syndrome. *J. Clin. Med.* **2018**, *7*, 191. [CrossRef]
13. Albouaini, K.; Egred, M.; Alahmar, A.; Wright, D.J. Cardiopulmonary exercise testing and its application. *Heart Br. Card. Soc.* **2007**, *93*, 1285–1292. [CrossRef]

14. Berger, M.; Kline, C.E.; Cepeda, F.X.; Rizzi, C.F.; Chapelle, C.; Laporte, S.; Hupin, D.; Raffin, J.; Costes, F.; Hargens, T.A.; et al. Does obstructive sleep apnea affect exercise capacity and the hemodynamic response to exercise? An individual patient data and aggregate meta-analysis. *Sleep Med. Rev.* **2019**, *45*, 42–53. [CrossRef]
15. Young, T.; Palta, M.; Dempsey, J.; Skatrud, J.; Weber, S.; Badr, S. The occurrence of sleep-disordered breathing among middle-aged adults. *N. Engl. J. Med.* **1993**, *328*, 1230–1235. [CrossRef]
16. Popovic, R.M.; White, D.P. Upper airway muscle activity in normal women: Influence of hormonal status. *J. Appl. Physiol.* **1998**, *84*, 1055–1062. [CrossRef] [PubMed]
17. Hou, Y.X.; Jia, S.S.; Liu, Y.H. 17β-Estradiol accentuates contractility of rat genioglossal muscle via regulation of estrogen receptor alpha. *Arch Oral. Biol.* **2010**, *55*, 309–317. [CrossRef] [PubMed]
18. Soriano-Co, M.; Vanhecke, T.E.; Franklin, B.A.; Sangal, R.B.; Hakmeh, B.; McCullough, P.A. Increased central adiposity in morbidly obese patients with obstructive sleep apnoea. *Intern. Med. J.* **2011**, *41*, 560–566. [CrossRef] [PubMed]
19. Trinder, J.; Kay, A.; Kleiman, J.; Dunai, J. Gender differences in airway resistance during sleep. *J Appl. Physiol.* **1997**, *83*, 1986–1997. [CrossRef]
20. Lin, C.M.; Davidson, T.M.; Ancoli-Israel, S. Gender differences in obstructive sleep apnea and treatment implications. *Sleep Med. Rev.* **2008**, *12*, 481–496. [CrossRef]
21. Tapan, Ö.O.; Sevinç, C.; İtil, B.O.; Öztura, İ.; Kayatekin, B.M.; Demiral, Y. Effect of Nasal Continuous Positive Airway Pressure Therapy on the Functional Respiratory Parameters and Cardiopulmonary Exercise Test in Obstructive Sleep Apnea Syndrome. *Turk. Thorac. J.* **2016**, *17*, 1–6. [CrossRef]
22. Przybyłowski, T.; Bielicki, P.; Kumor, M.; Hildebrand, K.; Maskey-Warzechowska, M.; Korczyński, P.; Chazan, R. Exercise capacity in patients with obstructive sleep apnea syndrome. *J. Physiol. Pharmacol. Off. J. Pol. Physiol. Soc.* **2007**, *58*, 563–574.
23. Cintra, F.D.; Tufik, S.; de Paola, A.; Feres, M.C.; Melo-Fujita, L.; Oliveira, W.; Rizzi, C.; Poyares, D. Cardiovascular profile in patients with obstructive sleep apnea. *Arq. Bras. Cardiol.* **2011**, *96*, 293–299. [CrossRef] [PubMed]
24. Kaleth, A.S.; Chittenden, T.W.; Hawkins, B.J.; Hargens, T.A.; Guill, S.G.; Zedalis, D.; Gregg, J.M.; Herbert, W.G. Unique cardiopulmonary exercise test responses in overweight middle-aged adults with obstructive sleep apnea. *Sleep Med.* **2007**, *8*, 160–168. [CrossRef]
25. Vanhecke, T.E.; Franklin, B.A.; Zalesin, K.C.; Sangal, R.B.; deJong, A.T.; Agrawal, V.; McCullough, P.A. Cardiorespiratory Fitness and Obstructive Sleep Apnea Syndrome in Morbidly Obese Patients. *Chest* **2008**, *134*, 539–545. [CrossRef]
26. Rizzi, C.F.; Cintra, F.; Mello-Fujita, L.; Rios, L.F.; Mendonca, E.T.; Feres, M.C.; Tufik, S.; Poyares, D. Does obstructive sleep apnea impair the cardiopulmonary response to exercise? *Sleep* **2013**, *36*, 547–553. [CrossRef]
27. Rizzi, C.F.; Cintra, F.; Risso, T.; Pulz, C.; Tufik, S.; de Paola, A.; Poyares, D. Exercise capacity and obstructive sleep apnea in lean subjects. *Chest* **2010**, *137*, 109–114. [CrossRef]
28. Powell, T.A.; Mysliwiec, V.; Aden, J.K.; Morris, M.J. Moderate to Severe Obstructive Sleep Apnea in Military Personnel Is Not Associated With Decreased Exercise Capacity. *J. Clin. Sleep Med. JCSM Off. Pub. Am. Acad. Sleep Med.* **2019**, *15*, 823–829. [CrossRef]
29. Mendelson, M.; Marillier, M.; Bailly, S.; Flore, P.; Borel, J.-C.; Vivodtzev, I.; Doutreleau, S.; Tamisier, R.; Pépin, J.-L.; Verges, S. Maximal exercise capacity in patients with obstructive sleep apnoea syndrome: A systematic review and meta-analysis. *Eur. Respir. J.* **2018**, *51*, 1702697. [CrossRef]
30. Beitler, J.R.; Awad, K.M.; Bakker, J.P.; Edwards, B.A.; DeYoung, P.; Djonlagic, I.; Forman, D.E.; Quan, S.F.; Malhotra, A. Obstructive sleep apnea is associated with impaired exercise capacity: A cross-sectional study. *J. Clin. Sleep Med. JCSM Off. Pub. Am. Acad. Sleep Med.* **2014**, *10*, 1199–1204. [CrossRef]
31. Lin, C.-C.; Lin, C.-K.; Wu, K.-M.; Chou, C.-S. Effect of treatment by nasal CPAP on cardiopulmonary exercise test in obstructive sleep apnea syndrome. *Lung* **2004**, *182*, 199–212. [CrossRef] [PubMed]
32. Maeder, M.T.; Ammann, P.; Münzer, T.; Schoch, O.D.; Korte, W.; Hürny, C.; Myers, J.; Rickli, H. Continuous positive airway pressure improves exercise capacity and heart rate recovery in obstructive sleep apnea. *Int. J. Cardiol.* **2009**, *132*, 75–83. [CrossRef] [PubMed]
33. Quadri, F.; Boni, E.; Pini, L.; Bottone, D.; Venturoli, N.; Corda, L.; Tantucci, C. Exercise tolerance in obstructive sleep apnea-hypopnea (OSAH), before and after CPAP treatment: Effects of autonomic dysfunction improvement. *Respir. Physiol. Neurobiol.* **2017**, *236*, 51–56. [CrossRef] [PubMed]

34. Ozsarac, I.; Bayram, N.; Uyar, M.; Kosovali, D.; Gundogdu, N.; Filiz, A. Effects of positive airway pressure therapy on exercise parameters in obstructive sleep apnea. *Ann. Saudi Med.* **2014**, *34*, 302–307. [CrossRef] [PubMed]
35. Kunos, L.; Lazar, Z.; Martinovszky, F.; Tarnoki, A.D.; Tarnoki, D.L.; Kovacs, D.; Forgo, B.; Horvath, P.; Losonczy, G.; Bikov, A. Overnight Changes in Lung Function of Obese Patients with Obstructive Sleep Apnoea. *Lung* **2017**, *195*, 127–133. [CrossRef]

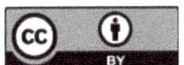

© 2020 by the authors. Licensee MDPI, Basel, Switzerland. This article is an open access article distributed under the terms and conditions of the Creative Commons Attribution (CC BY) license (http://creativecommons.org/licenses/by/4.0/).

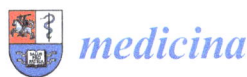

Article

Circulating Soluble Urokinase-Type Plasminogen Activator Receptor in Obstructive Sleep Apnoea

Renata Marietta Bocskei [1,2], Martina Meszaros [1], Adam Domonkos Tarnoki [3], David Laszlo Tarnoki [3], Laszlo Kunos [1], Zsofia Lazar [1] and Andras Bikov [1,4,*]

1. Department of Pulmonology, Semmelweis University, 1083 Budapest, Hungary; drbocskeirenata@gmail.com (R.M.B.); martina.meszaros1015@gmail.com (M.M.); laszlokunos@gmail.com (L.K.); lazar.zsofia@med.semmelweis-univ.hu (Z.L.)
2. Department of Pulmonology, Szent Borbala County Hospital, 2800 Tatabánya, Hungary
3. Medical Imaging Centre, Semmelweis University, 1082 Budapest, Hungary; tarnoki2@gmail.com (A.D.T.); tarnoki4@gmail.com (D.L.T.)
4. North West Lung Centre, Manchester University NHS Foundation Trust, Manchester M23 9LT, UK
* Correspondence: andras.bikov@gmail.com; Tel.: +36-203-141-599

Received: 4 January 2020; Accepted: 5 February 2020; Published: 14 February 2020

Abstract: *Background and Objectives*: Obstructive sleep apnoea (OSA) is associated with heightened systemic inflammation and a hypercoagulation state. Soluble urokinase-type plasminogen activator receptor (suPAR) plays a role in fibrinolysis and systemic inflammation. However, suPAR has not been investigated in OSA. *Materials and Methods*: A total of 53 patients with OSA and 15 control volunteers participated in the study. Medical history was taken and in-hospital sleep studies were performed. Plasma suPAR levels were determined by ELISA. *Results*: There was no difference in plasma suPAR values between patients with OSA (2.198 ± 0.675 ng/mL) and control subjects (2.088 ± 0.976 ng/mL, $p = 0.62$). Neither was there any difference when patients with OSA were divided into mild (2.134 ± 0.799 ng/mL), moderate (2.274 ± 0.597 ng/mL) and severe groups (2.128 ± 0.744 ng/mL, $p = 0.84$). There was no significant correlation between plasma suPAR and indices of OSA severity, blood results or comorbidities, such as hypertension, diabetes, dyslipidaemia or cardiovascular disease. Plasma suPAR levels were higher in women when all subjects were analysed together (2.487 ± 0.683 vs. 1.895 ± 0.692 ng/mL, $p < 0.01$), and also separately in controls (2.539 ± 0.956 vs. 1.411 ± 0.534 ng/mL, $p = 0.02$) and patients (2.467 ± 0.568 vs. 1.991 ± 0.686 ng/mL, $p < 0.01$). *Conclusions*: Our results suggest that suPAR does not play a significant role in the pathophysiology of OSA. The significant gender difference needs to be considered when conducting studies on circulating suPAR.

Keywords: biomarkers; fibrinolysis; inflammation; OSAHS; sleep disordered breathing

1. Introduction

Obstructive sleep apnoea (OSA) is a common disease which is characterised by repetitive collapse of the upper airways during sleep which results in intermittent hypoxia and frequent microarousals. These processes lead to the development of cardiometabolic comorbidities, such as hypertension, cardiovascular disease, diabetes and dyslipidaemia, which frequently accompany OSA.

Chronic intermittent hypoxia and increased sympathetic tone induce production of pro-inflammatory molecules, such as interleukin (IL)-6, IL-1β, tumour necrosis factor-α [1] or complement elements [2] and suppresses the release of anti-inflammatory [3,4] molecules. Linked to inflammation and sympathetic activity, OSA is characterised by a hypercoagulation state [5–9]. Accelerated systemic inflammation and increased coagulation may contribute to the development of cardiovascular disease and acute cardiovascular events [10].

Soluble urokinase-type plasminogen activator receptor (suPAR) is a molecule which plays a role in both inflammation and coagulation. It is produced upon cleavage of the membrane-bound urokinase-type plasminogen activator receptor (uPAR). The cleavage is facilitated by urokinase-type plasminogen activator (uPA), plasmin, matrix metalloproteases, neutrophil elastase and cathepsin G [11]. The urokinase receptor (also known as uPAR) is expressed by endothelial cells, macrophages, monocytes, neutrophils, lymphocytes, smooth muscle cells and fibroblasts [12,13]. It is upregulated under infections and as an effect of pro-inflammatory cytokines [11,13–15], while suPAR contributes to plasminogen activation, cell adhesion, chemotaxis and immune cell activation [16]. However, uPAR also acts as a scavenger receptor for uPA, inhibiting its actions [17]. In large studies, plasma suPAR was elevated in coronary artery disease and cerebrovascular disease and correlated with their severity and cardiovascular mortality [18–20]. Higher suPAR levels were also observed in obesity [21], which is the main etiological factor for OSA in the Western population [22].

Only one study has investigated suPAR in probable OSA so far [23]. Patients were categorised to high and low-risk OSA based on the Berlin questionnaire and neck circumferences; however, no objective sleep tests were performed. In this study, there was a tendency for higher suPAR levels in the high-risk group, but the difference did not reach a significant level [23].

We hypothesised that circulating suPAR concentrations are elevated in OSA compared to health and probably relate to disease severity. The aim of the study was to investigate these using standardised diagnostic tests.

2. Materials and Methods

2.1. Study Design and Subjects

We recruited 68 volunteers (54 ± 13 years, 36 men) who were referred for a sleep study to the Sleep Unit, Department of Pulmonology, Semmelweis University due to suspected OSA (i.e., snoring, daytime tiredness, obesity, comorbidities). After giving informed consent, medical history was taken and patients filled out the ESS, which was followed by in-laboratory cardiorespiratory polygraphy ($n = 20$) or polysomnography ($n = 48$). In the morning, blood pressure was measured; fasting venous blood was taken for lipid profile, glucose, creatinine, C-reactive protein (CRP) and suPAR measurements between 6:00 and 8:00 a.m. Glomerular filtration rate (GFR) was calculated using the Modification of Diet in Renal Disease equation.

Comorbidities were defined according to the participants' report, available medical records, medications, morning blood pressures and fasting blood laboratory results. In detail, hypertension was excluded if there was no history for high blood pressure. Participants did not take anti-hypertensive medications, and morning blood pressure was within the normal range. In line with this, diabetes and dyslipidaemia were excluded if there was no history for these comorbidities, participants did not take antidiabetic or anti-dyslipidaemia medications, and the fasting blood glucose and lipid results were in the normal range. Cardiovascular disease was excluded based on absence of symptoms and negative medical history.

2.2. Sleep Studies

Inpatient polysomnography and cardiorespiratory polygraphy were performed as described previously [2–4] using Somnoscreen Plus Tele PSG (Somnomedics GMBH Germany). Sleep stages, movements and cardiopulmonary events were scored manually according to the American Academy of Sleep Medicine [24] guidelines. Apnoea was defined as a 90% airflow decrease, which lasted for more than 10 s, and hypopnoea was defined as at least 30% airflow decrease lasting for at least 10 s, which was related to a ≥3% oxygen desideration or an arousal. Total sleep time (TST), sleep period time (SPT), total sleep time spent with oxygen saturation below 90% (TST90%) and minimal oxygen saturation (minSatO$_2$) were recorded, and apnoea–hypopnoea index (AHI), oxygen desaturation index

(ODI) and arousal index (AI) were calculated. Obstructive sleep apnoea was defined as having an AHI ≥ 5/h.

2.3. SuPAR Measurements

Venous blood was taken into EDTA tubes. Within 30 minutes, blood samples were centrifuged at 4 °C for 10 min at 1500 rpm, and the plasma was stored at −80 °C until further analysis. Plasma suPAR levels were measured using a commercially available ELISA kit (ViroGates A/S, Birkerød, Denmark) as described previously [25]. The samples were measured in duplicates, and the mean concentration was used. The intra-assay coefficient of variation was 9 ± 11% with a lower limit of detection of 0.1 ng/mL. All suPAR concentrations were above the detection limit.

2.4. Statistical Analyses

Statistica 12 (StatSoft, Inc., Tulsa, OK, USA) was used for statistical analyses. The normality of the data was checked with the Kolmogorov–Smirnov test, which showed normal distribution for suPAR concentrations. Patient and control groups were compared with unpaired t-test, Mann–Whitney, Chi-square and Fisher tests. Plasma suPAR was related to clinical and demographic variables using linear and logistic regression and compared among different OSA severities with general mixed linear models. These analyses were repeated following adjustment for age, gender, body mass index (BMI), type of the sleep tests, anticoagulant and antithrombotic medications and GFR as well. To avoid the confounding effect of hypertension and diabetes, OSA and control groups were compared when subjects affected by these comorbidities were excluded. A p value <0.05 was considered significant. The suPAR results are presented as mean ± standard deviation with 95% confidence intervals.

The minimal sample size was estimated to detect differences in plasma suPAR levels between the OSA and control groups with an effect size of 0.80, power of 0.80 and alpha of 0.05 [26]. These numbers were based on a distribution of plasma suPAR values in control subjects [25]. Post-hoc sensitivity analyses ensured it was possible to detect correlations between suPAR and clinical variables within −0.23 and 0.23, minimal and maximal critical r values, statistical power of 0.80 and alpha of 0.05 [26].

The study was approved by the Semmelweis University Ethics Committee (TUKEB 30/2014 and 172/2018, approved on 26 October 2018) and was conducted according to the Declaration of Helsinki. Patients provided their written consent.

3. Results

3.1. Patient Characteristics

OSA was diagnosed in 53 cases (6 mild, 25 moderate and 22 severe; AHI 5–14.9/h, 15–29.9/h and ≥30/h, respectively). Patients with OSA had higher BMI, systolic (SBP) and diastolic blood pressure (DBP), AHI, ODI, SPT, TST, TST 90% and lower high density lipoprotein cholesterol (HDL-C) and MinSatO$_2$ compared to controls (all $p < 0.05$, Table 1). In addition, patients with OSA tended to be older ($p = 0.08$) and sleepier ($p = 0.05$), and the prevalence of dyslipidaemia tended to be higher in OSA ($p = 0.07$, Table 1).

Table 1. Subjects' characteristics *.

	Control (n = 15)	OSA (n = 53)	Total (n = 68)	p
Age (years)	48/31–62/	59/49–64/	54.6/44–64/	0.08
Male (n, %)	6, 40%	30, 57%	36, 53%	0.26
BMI (kg/m^2)	24.6±4.58	32.37±5.66	30.66±6.31	<0.01
Hypertension (%)	33	70	62	0.01
Diabetes (%)	0	13	10	0.14
Dyslipidaemia (%)	27	53	47	0.07
Cardiovascular disease (%)	13	11	12	0.83

Table 1. Cont.

	Control (n = 15)	OSA (n = 53)	Total (n = 68)	p
Cardiac arrhythmia (%)	13	26	24	0.29
Smokers (%)	20	23	22	0.83
Subjects taking anticoagulants (%)	0	11	10	0.32
Subjects taking antithrombotic drugs (%)	13	11	12	1.00
SBP (mmHg)	120/118–131/	138/130–150/	132/120–140/	**<0.01**
DBP (mmHg)	70/70–75/	85/76–90/	80/70–90/	**<0.01**
Creatinine (mmol/L)	77.5/66.3–83.5/	66/61–79/	70.0/62.0–82.5/	0.17
GFR (mL/min/1.73m^2)	82.26±15.17	88.37±17.91	86.75±17.3	0.26
CRP (mg/L)	2.34/0.92–3.95/	3.0/1.36–4.65/	3.0/1.33–4.48/	0.23
Glucose (mmol/L)	4.65/4.1–5.3/	5.2/4.8–6.1/	5.1/4.7–5.7/	0.05
Cholesterol (mmol/L)	5.91±1.04	5.33±1.13	5.46±1.13	0.08
HDL-C (mmol/L)	1.84/1.58–2.34/	1.28/1.06–1.62/	1.36/1.17–1.82/	**<0.01**
LDL-C (mmol/L)	3.41±0.89	3.16±1.02	3.22±0.99	0.39
Triglyceride (mmol/L)	1.23/0.94–1.32/	1.33/1.07–1.97/	1.28/1.04–1.92/	0.10
Lipoprotein (a) (mmol/L)	0.2/0.0–0.4/	0.17/0.10–0.49/	0.18/0.07–0.44/	0.56
AHI (1/h)	1.6/1.0–2.4/	27.5/18.55–42.75/	21.89/8.9–40.63/	**<0.01**
ODI (1/h)	0.9/0.4–1.7/	23.2/14.1–38.95/	19.65/6.2–32/	**<0.01**
SPT (min)	395.19±36.1	439.93±72.82	427.81±67.62	**0.04**
TST (min)	398/319–409.5/	428/384.5–452/	410.5/363.25–440.75/	**<0.01**
TST90% (%)	0.0/0.0–0.1/	6/1.7–12.5/	3.85/0.4–11.6/	**<0.01**
Minimal oxygen saturation (%)	91/88.25–92.75/	82.5/76.8–85/	83/77.8–88/	**<0.01**
ESS	5.0/2.75–7.0/	7/5–10/	6/4–8/ 6.6±3.68	0.05

* Data are presented as mean ± standard deviation or median/25%–75% percentile/. Significant differences are highlighted in bold. AHI—apnoea–hypopnoea index, BMI—body mass index, DBP—diastolic blood pressure, CRP—C-reactive protein, ESS—Epworth Sleepiness Scale, GFR—glomerular filtration rate, HDL-C—high density lipoprotein cholesterol, LDL-C—low density lipoprotein cholesterol, ODI—oxygen desaturation index, SBP—systolic blood pressure, SPT—sleep period time, TST—total sleep time, TST90%—total sleep time spent with oxygen saturation below 90%.

3.2. Circulating suPAR Results

There was no difference in plasma suPAR concentrations between the controls (2.088 ± 0.976/1.548–2.628/ ng/mL) and patients with OSA (2.198 ± 0.675/2.012–2.384/ ng/mL, unadjusted $p = 0.62$, $p = 0.99$ after adjustment, Figure 1). Similarly, there was no difference between mild (2.134 ± 0.799/1.295–2.974/ ng/mL), moderate (2.274 ± 0.597/2.028–2.521/ ng/mL) and severe patients (2.128 ± 0.744/1.798–2.458/ ng/mL, unadjusted $p = 0.84$, $p = 0.78$ after adjustment, Figure 2). In line with this, there was no relationship between plasma suPAR levels and AHI ($p = 0.65$), ODI ($p = 0.58$), TST90% ($p = 0.35$), minSatO$_2$ ($p = 0.16$), AI ($p = 0.38$), TST ($p = 0.60$), SPT ($p = 0.41$) or ESS ($p = 0.44$). We noted two outliers in the control group. These subjects did not differ in their demographics or clinical characteristics from other controls. Excluding them from analyses resulted in tendency for higher suPAR levels in OSA ($p = 0.050$); however, after adjustment for covariates this difference was not significant ($p = 0.259$).

Plasma suPAR directly correlated with age when all subjects were analysed together (r = 0.33, $p < 0.01$), or when patients with OSA were investigated separately (r = 0.30, $p = 0.02$). However, when adjusting for covariates, these correlations were no longer significant (both $p > 0.05$).

Plasma suPAR levels were higher in women when all subjects were analysed together (2.487 ± 0.683/2.241–2.733/ vs. 1.895 ± 0.692/2.221–2.713/ ng/mL, $p < 0.01$, in controls (2.539 ± 0.956/1.804–3.474/ vs. 1.411 ± 0.534/0.851–1.971/ ng/mL, $p = 0.02$) and in OSA (2.467 ± 0.568/2.221–2.713/ vs. 1.991 ± 0.686/1.735–2.247/ ng/mL, $p < 0.01$, Figure 3). These intergender differences remained significant even after adjustment for covariates. Due to the asymmetric gender distribution in the OSA and control groups, plasma suPAR levels were compared in control and OSA women and men separately. There was no difference in women (2.467 ± 0.568/2.221–2.713/ vs. 2.539 ± 0.956/1.804–3.474/ ng/mL, OSA vs. controls, $p = 0.79$). However, plasma suPAR tended to be higher in male patients with OSA (1.991 ± 0.686/1.735–2.247/ ng/mL, n = 30) compared to controls (1.411 ± 0.534/0.851–1.971/ ng/mL, n = 6,

$p = 0.059$). Despite this potential signal, there was no relationship between AHI and suPAR levels in either men or women (both $p > 0.05$).

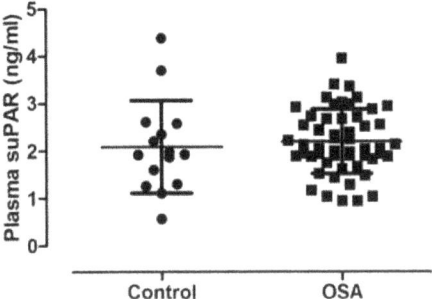

Figure 1. Comparison of plasma soluble urokinase-type plasminogen activator receptor (suPAR) levels between patients with OSA and controls. There was no difference between the two groups in plasma suPAR levels ($p = 0.62$). Mean ± standard deviation is presented.

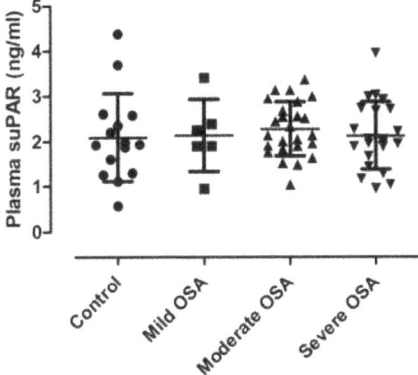

Figure 2. Comparison of plasma suPAR levels among different disease severities. There was no difference among the groups in plasma suPAR levels ($p = 0.87$). Mean ± standard deviation is presented.

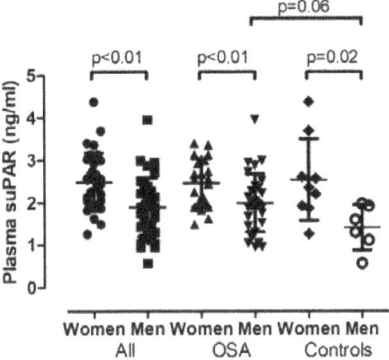

Figure 3. Comparison of plasma suPAR levels between women and men. Plasma suPAR levels were higher in women in patients with OSA, in controls and when the subjects were analysed together. Mean ± standard deviation is presented.

Patients with OSA who took anticoagulants had higher plasma suPAR levels (2.739 ± 0.547/2.164–3.313/ vs. 2.129 ± 0.663/1.934–2.323/ ng/mL, $p = 0.03$); however, this difference became insignificant after adjusting for covariates ($p>0.05$). None of the other correlations between plasma suPAR concentrations, demographics, clinical variables or comorbidities, such as hypertension, diabetes, dyslipidaemia or cardiovascular disease were significant in any of the studied groups (all $p>0.05$).

3.3. Plasma suPAR Results in Control and OSA Participants without Hypertension or Diabetes

There was no difference in plasma suPAR levels when controls without hypertension (1.903 ± 0.922/1.244–2.562/ ng/mL, $n = 10$) were compared to OSA patients without hypertension (2.110 ± 0.671/1.753–2.467/ ng/mL, $n = 16$, $p = 0.51$). Similarly, no difference was found between controls without diabetes (2.088 ± 0.976/1.548–2.628/ ng/mL, $n = 15$) and OSA patients without diabetes (2.203 ± 0.676/2.002-2.403/, $n = 46$, $p = 0.61$). In line with this, there was no difference when controls without hypertension and diabetes (1.903 ± 0.922/1.244–2.562/ ng/mL, $n = 10$) were compared to OSA patients without hypertension and diabetes (2.165 ± 0.656/1.802–2.528/ ng/mL, $n = 15$, $p = 0.41$).

4. Discussion

In the current study, we analysed plasma suPAR levels in OSA, but did not find any difference compared to controls, nor did suPAR concentrations correlate with disease severity. This implies that suPAR may not play a significant role in the pathophysiology of OSA; however, due to the small number of controls and the significant gender effect on suPAR levels, our results must be interpreted carefully.

Obstructive sleep apnoea is associated with heightened systemic inflammation, theoretically contributing to higher uPAR expression [11,13–15]. However, the cleavage of uPAR may be slower in OSA due to decreased levels of uPA [8] and plasmin [5,6,23]. The expression of uPA is induced by female sexual hormones [20] and the proto-oncogenic survivin [27], which presented decreased expressions in OSA [3,28]. Plasmin is formed by plasminogen, and this reaction is blocked by plasminogen activator-inhibitors (PAI), shown to be upregulated in OSA [5,6,23]. In addition, OSA is associated with decreased levels of transforming growth factor-β [8], an inducer of uPAR transcription [29,30]. These studies suggest that although uPAR expression may be upregulated by systemic inflammation in OSA [11,13–15]; this is counterbalanced by the reduced cleavage.

It has been shown that plasma suPAR levels are higher in women [20] and related to BMI and waist circumference only in females [20]. In addition, plasma suPAR levels were prognostic for cardiovascular events only in women [19] and more strongly related to coronary artery calcification in women than in men [31]. Our results are in line with the previous findings [20], namely that suPAR was higher in women in both OSA and controls. A potential reason for the gender differences is that uPA is released upon stimulation by progesterone and oestradiol [32] resulting in higher uPAR cleavage. Female sexual hormones are protective in OSA [33], contributing to male predominance in sleep apnoea [33,34]. To exclude this effect, analyses were performed after adjustment for gender and suPAR was compared between OSA and controls in women and men separately. Although there was a tendency for higher suPAR levels in men in OSA, there was no relationship with OSA severity in males. Of note, the number of men in the control group was small, and these analyses were underpowered. Nevertheless, this difference could be a potential signal which should be investigated in further studies. We believe that our current results would provide basis for further study design. In line with the previous findings [35], plasma suPAR levels were directly related to age; however, this correlation disappeared after adjustment for covariates. Although higher suPAR levels were associated with obesity [21], this has not been confirmed by the current study.

Our study has limitations. First, the sample size, especially in the control group, was low. This could have potentially led to type II error, especially due to significant difference in age, gender and comorbidity distribution. To avoid this, our analyses were adjusted on potential confounders. The plasma suPAR levels were not different between patients with OSA and controls either in unadjusted or adjusted comparisons. Still, our results should be interpreted carefully, especially considering the exclusion of the two outliers which resulted in differences between the two groups. The sample size calculations were based on our previous study [25], showing higher suPAR levels in COPD. Although the number of participants may seem low, it may not be the likely reason for the lack of differences between OSA and controls considering the wide overlap of suPAR values between the two groups and the lack of significant relationship between markers of OSA severity and suPAR levels. In line with this, a second limitation is the unbalanced proportion of comorbidities in the OSA and control groups.

Elevated suPAR levels are associated with cardiovascular disease and diabetes [36]. OSA represents a risk for cardio metabolic disease [22], which was reflected in the asymmetric proportion of comorbidities in the OSA and control groups. However, we did not find any relationship between plasma suPAR concentrations and comorbidities. To further evaluate this, we performed additional analyses in participants without hypertension or diabetes. We did not find any difference in plasma suPAR values between controls and patients with OSA in non-hypertensive or nondiabetic volunteers. Of note, the study has not been powered to address this question. We believe our results could provide a basis to design further studies involving groups balanced on the profile of comorbidities. The third limitation is that although patients represented a large range of OSA severity, in average, they were minimally symptomatic. It has recently been reported that patients with OSA and excessive daytime sleepiness have a higher risk for cardiovascular disease [37]. Inclusion of more symptomatic patients in studies investigating systemic inflammation is therefore warranted. The fourth limitation is the significant gender-effect which has been discussed above. The strengths of the study include the application of objective sleep tests, detailed characterisation of the studied population and robust methodology for plasma suPAR measurement.

Only one study has examined suPAR in possible OSA. Von Kanel et al. divided 329 South African teachers based on their response to the Berlin questionnaire and/or neck circumference into a high-risk and low-risk OSA group. Most notably, no objective sleep study has been performed. Although the levels of fibrinogen and PAI-1 were elevated together with slower clot lysis time, there was only a tendency for higher suPAR levels in the high-risk group [23]. The Berlin questionnaire is a moderately sensitive, but not specific screening tool for OSA [38]; therefore, these results must be interpreted carefully. Nevertheless, the previous [23] and the current findings indicate that hyper-coagulation in OSA is driven by high fibrin formation, reduced plasminogen activation by increased PAI-1 and lower uPA without a significant difference in the uPAR signalling.

5. Conclusions

In conclusion, we did not find altered plasma suPAR levels in patients with OSA vs. controls. Our results suggest that this molecule does not play a significant role in hyper coagulation and accelerated systemic inflammation in OSA and cannot be applied as a readout signal for these pathophysiological processes. However, the significant gender differences are noteworthy and must be considered when designing future studies with suPAR.

Author Contributions: R.M.B. designed the study and acquired funding. M.M. performed ELISA measurements and sleep study analyses. A.D.T., D.L.T. and Z.L. participated in the design and contributed to recruiting and clinically characterising the patients. L.K. performed sleep study analyses. A.B. designed the study, drafted the manuscript and performed statistical and sleep study analyses. All authors read and approved the final manuscript.

Funding: The study was supported by Hungarian Respiratory Society grants to Andras Bikov and David L. Tarnoki as well as Semmelweis University grant to Laszlo Kunos. This publication was supported by the Janos Bolyai Research Scholarship of the Hungarian Academy of Sciences to Andras Bikov. Andras Bikov is supported by the NIHR Manchester BRC.

Acknowledgments: The authors are also grateful to Elektro-Oxigén Inc. for providing polysomnographic devices and Monika Banlaky for her assistance in sleep studies.

Conflicts of Interest: The authors state no conflict of interest. The funders had no role in the design of the study, collection, analyses, interpretation of data, writing of the manuscript or the decision to publish the results.

References

1. Kent, B.D.; Ryan, S.; McNicholas, W.T. Obstructive sleep apnea and inflammation: Relationship to cardiovascular co-morbidity. *Respir. Physiol. Neurobiol.* **2011**, *178*, 475–481. [CrossRef] [PubMed]
2. Horvath, P.; Tarnoki, D.L.; Tarnoki, A.D.; Karlinger, K.; Lazar, Z.; Losonczy, G.; Kunos, L.; Bikov, A. Complement system activation in obstructive sleep apnea. *J. Sleep Res.* **2018**, *27*, e12674. [CrossRef] [PubMed]
3. Kunos, L.; Horvath, P.; Kis, A.; Tarnoki, D.L.; Tarnoki, A.D.; Lazar, Z.; Bikov, A. Circulating Survivin Levels in Obstructive Sleep Apnoea. *Lung* **2018**, *196*, 417–424. [CrossRef] [PubMed]
4. Pako, J.; Kunos, L.; Meszaros, M.; Tarnoki, D.L.; Tarnoki, A.D.; Horvath, I.; Bikov, A. Decreased Levels of Anti-Aging Klotho in Obstructive Sleep Apnea. *Rejuvenation Res.* **2019**. [CrossRef]
5. Bagai, K.; Muldowney, J.A., 3rd; Song, Y.; Wang, L.; Bagai, J.; Artibee, K.J.; Vaughan, D.E.; Malow, B.A. Circadian variability of fibrinolytic markers and endothelial function in patients with obstructive sleep apnea. *Sleep* **2014**, *37*, 359–367. [CrossRef]
6. Zakrzewski, M.; Zakrzewska, E.; Kicinski, P.; Przybylska-Kuc, S.; Dybala, A.; Myslinski, W.; Pastryk, J.; Tomaszewski, T.; Mosiewicz, J. Evaluation of Fibrinolytic Inhibitors: Alpha-2-Antiplasmin and Plasminogen Activator Inhibitor 1 in Patients with Obstructive Sleep Apnoea. *PLoS ONE* **2016**, *11*, e0166725. [CrossRef]
7. Robinson, G.V.; Pepperell, J.C.; Segal, H.C.; Davies, R.J.; Stradling, J.R. Circulating cardiovascular risk factors in obstructive sleep apnoea: Data from randomised controlled trials. *Thorax* **2004**, *59*, 777–782. [CrossRef]
8. Steffanina, A.; Proietti, L.; Antonaglia, C.; Palange, P.; Angelici, E.; Canipari, R. The Plasminogen System and Transforming Growth Factor-beta in Subjects With Obstructive Sleep Apnea Syndrome: Effects of CPAP Treatment. *Respir. Care* **2015**, *60*, 1643–1651. [CrossRef]
9. Garcia-Ortega, A.; Manas, E.; Lopez-Reyes, R.; Selma, M.J.; Garcia-Sanchez, A.; Oscullo, G.; Jimenez, D.; Martinez-Garcia, M.A. Obstructive sleep apnoea and venous thromboembolism: Pathophysiological links and clinical implications. *Eur. Respir. J.* **2019**, *53*. [CrossRef]
10. Kohler, M.; Stradling, J.R. Mechanisms of vascular damage in obstructive sleep apnea. *Nat. Rev. Cardiol.* **2010**, *7*, 677–685. [CrossRef]
11. Enocsson, H.; Sjowall, C.; Wettero, J. Soluble urokinase plasminogen activator receptor—A valuable biomarker in systemic lupus erythematosus? *Clin. Chim. Acta Int. J. Clin. Chem.* **2015**, *444*, 234–241. [CrossRef] [PubMed]
12. Donadello, K.; Scolletta, S.; Covajes, C.; Vincent, J.L. suPAR as a prognostic biomarker in sepsis. *BMC Med.* **2012**, *10*, 2. [CrossRef] [PubMed]
13. Thuno, M.; Macho, B.; Eugen-Olsen, J. suPAR: The molecular crystal ball. *Dis. Markers* **2009**, *27*, 157–172. [CrossRef] [PubMed]
14. Nykjaer, A.; Moller, B.; Todd, R.F., 3rd; Christensen, T.; Andreasen, P.A.; Gliemann, J.; Petersen, C.M. Urokinase receptor. An activation antigen in human T lymphocytes. *J. Immunol. (Baltim. Md. 1950)* **1994**, *152*, 505–516.
15. Chavakis, T.; Willuweit, A.K.; Lupu, F.; Preissner, K.T.; Kanse, S.M. Release of soluble urokinase receptor from vascular cells. *Thromb. Haemost.* **2001**, *86*, 686–693. [CrossRef] [PubMed]
16. Eugen-Olsen, J. suPAR—A future risk marker in bacteremia. *J. Intern. Med.* **2011**, *270*, 29–31. [CrossRef]
17. Masucci, M.T.; Pedersen, N.; Blasi, F. A soluble, ligand binding mutant of the human urokinase plasminogen activator receptor. *J. Biol. Chem.* **1991**, *266*, 8655–8658.
18. Eapen, D.J.; Manocha, P.; Ghasemzadeh, N.; Patel, R.S.; Al Kassem, H.; Hammadah, M.; Veledar, E.; Le, N.A.; Pielak, T.; Thorball, C.W.; et al. Soluble urokinase plasminogen activator receptor level is an independent predictor of the presence and severity of coronary artery disease and of future adverse events. *J. Am. Heart Assoc.* **2014**, *3*, e001118. [CrossRef]
19. Diederichsen, M.Z.; Diederichsen, S.Z.; Mickley, H.; Steffensen, F.H.; Lambrechtsen, J.; Sand, N.P.R.; Christensen, K.L.; Olsen, M.H.; Diederichsen, A.; Gronhoj, M.H. Prognostic value of suPAR and hs-CRP on cardiovascular disease. *Atherosclerosis* **2018**, *271*, 245–251. [CrossRef]
20. Lyngbaek, S.; Sehestedt, T.; Marott, J.L.; Hansen, T.W.; Olsen, M.H.; Andersen, O.; Linneberg, A.; Madsbad, S.; Haugaard, S.B.; Eugen-Olsen, J.; et al. CRP and suPAR are differently related to anthropometry and subclinical organ damage. *Int. J. Cardiol.* **2013**, *167*, 781–785. [CrossRef]

21. Cancello, R.; Rouault, C.; Guilhem, G.; Bedel, J.F.; Poitou, C.; Di Blasio, A.M.; Basdevant, A.; Tordjman, J.; Clement, K. Urokinase plasminogen activator receptor in adipose tissue macrophages of morbidly obese subjects. *Obes. Facts* **2011**, *4*, 17–25. [CrossRef] [PubMed]
22. Peppard, P.E.; Young, T.; Barnet, J.H.; Palta, M.; Hagen, E.W.; Hla, K.M. Increased prevalence of sleep-disordered breathing in adults. *Am. J. Epidemiol.* **2013**, *177*, 1006–1014. [CrossRef] [PubMed]
23. von Kanel, R.; Malan, N.T.; Hamer, M.; Lambert, G.W.; Schlaich, M.; Reimann, M.; Malan, L. Three-year changes of prothrombotic factors in a cohort of South Africans with a high clinical suspicion of obstructive sleep apnea. *Thromb. Haemost.* **2016**, *115*, 63–72. [CrossRef] [PubMed]
24. Berry, R.B.; Budhiraja, R.; Gottlieb, D.J.; Gozal, D.; Iber, C.; Kapur, V.K.; Marcus, C.L.; Mehra, R.; Parthasarathy, S.; Quan, S.F.; et al. Rules for scoring respiratory events in sleep: Update of the 2007 AASM Manual for the Scoring of Sleep and Associated Events. Deliberations of the Sleep Apnea Definitions Task Force of the American Academy of Sleep Medicine. *J. Clin. Sleep Med. Off. Publ. Am. Acad. Sleep Med.* **2012**, *8*, 597–619. [CrossRef]
25. Bocskei, R.M.; Benczur, B.; Losonczy, G.; Illyes, M.; Cziraki, A.; Muller, V.; Bohacs, A.; Bikov, A. Soluble Urokinase-Type Plasminogen Activator Receptor and Arterial Stiffness in Patients with COPD. *Lung* **2019**, *197*, 189–197. [CrossRef] [PubMed]
26. Faul, F.; Erdfelder, E.; Buchner, A.; Lang, A.G. Statistical power analyses using G*Power 3.1: Tests for correlation and regression analyses. *Behav. Res. Methods* **2009**, *41*, 1149–1160. [CrossRef] [PubMed]
27. Baran, M.; Mollers, L.N.; Andersson, S.; Jonsson, I.M.; Ekwall, A.K.; Bjersing, J.; Tarkowski, A.; Bokarewa, M. Survivin is an essential mediator of arthritis interacting with urokinase signalling. *J. Cell. Mol. Med.* **2009**, *13*, 3797–3808. [CrossRef]
28. Stavaras, C.; Pastaka, C.; Papala, M.; Gravas, S.; Tzortzis, V.; Melekos, M.; Seitanidis, G.; Gourgoulianis, K.I. Sexual function in pre- and post-menopausal women with obstructive sleep apnea syndrome. *Int. J. Impot. Res.* **2012**, *24*, 228–233. [CrossRef]
29. Lund, L.R.; Ellis, V.; Ronne, E.; Pyke, C.; Dano, K. Transcriptional and post-transcriptional regulation of the receptor for urokinase-type plasminogen activator by cytokines and tumour promoters in the human lung carcinoma cell line A549. *Biochem. J.* **1995**, *310*, 345–352. [CrossRef]
30. Shetty, S.; Idell, S. A urokinase receptor mRNA binding protein from rabbit lung fibroblasts and mesothelial cells. *Am. J. Physiol.* **1998**, *274*, L871–L882. [CrossRef]
31. Sorensen, M.H.; Gerke, O.; Eugen-Olsen, J.; Munkholm, H.; Lambrechtsen, J.; Sand, N.P.; Mickley, H.; Rasmussen, L.M.; Olsen, M.H.; Diederichsen, A. Soluble urokinase plasminogen activator receptor is in contrast to high-sensitive C-reactive-protein associated with coronary artery calcifications in healthy middle-aged subjects. *Atherosclerosis* **2014**, *237*, 60–66. [CrossRef]
32. Guan, Y.M.; Carlberg, M.; Bruse, C.; Carlstrom, K.; Bergqvist, A. Effects of hormones on uPA, PAI-1 and suPAR from cultured endometrial and ovarian endometriotic stromal cells. *Acta Obstet. Gynecol. Scand.* **2002**, *81*, 389–397. [CrossRef] [PubMed]
33. Lin, C.M.; Davidson, T.M.; Ancoli-Israel, S. Gender differences in obstructive sleep apnea and treatment implications. *Sleep Med. Rev.* **2008**, *12*, 481–496. [CrossRef] [PubMed]
34. Tsai, M.S.; Lee, L.A.; Tsai, Y.T.; Yang, Y.H.; Liu, C.Y.; Lin, M.H.; Hsu, C.M.; Chen, C.K.; Li, H.Y. Sleep apnea and risk of vertigo: A nationwide population-based cohort study. *Laryngoscope* **2018**, *128*, 763–768. [CrossRef] [PubMed]
35. Andersen, O.; Eugen-Olsen, J.; Kofoed, K.; Iversen, J.; Haugaard, S.B. Soluble urokinase plasminogen activator receptor is a marker of dysmetabolism in HIV-infected patients receiving highly active antiretroviral therapy. *J. Med Virol.* **2008**, *80*, 209–216. [CrossRef] [PubMed]
36. Eugen-Olsen, J.; Andersen, O.; Linneberg, A.; Ladelund, S.; Hansen, T.W.; Langkilde, A.; Petersen, J.; Pielak, T.; Moller, L.N.; Jeppesen, J.; et al. Circulating soluble urokinase plasminogen activator receptor predicts cancer, cardiovascular disease, diabetes and mortality in the general population. *J. Intern. Med.* **2010**, *268*, 296–308. [CrossRef] [PubMed]

37. Mazzotti, D.R.; Keenan, B.T.; Lim, D.C.; Gottlieb, D.J.; Kim, J.; Pack, A.I. Symptom Subtypes of Obstructive Sleep Apnea Predict Incidence of Cardiovascular Outcomes. *Am. J. Respir. Crit. Care Med.* **2019**, *200*, 493–506. [CrossRef] [PubMed]
38. Chiu, H.Y.; Chen, P.Y.; Chuang, L.P.; Chen, N.H.; Tu, Y.K.; Hsieh, Y.J.; Wang, Y.C.; Guilleminault, C. Diagnostic accuracy of the Berlin questionnaire, STOP-BANG, STOP, and Epworth sleepiness scale in detecting obstructive sleep apnea: A bivariate meta-analysis. *Sleep Med. Rev.* **2017**, *36*, 57–70. [CrossRef]

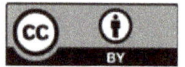

© 2020 by the authors. Licensee MDPI, Basel, Switzerland. This article is an open access article distributed under the terms and conditions of the Creative Commons Attribution (CC BY) license (http://creativecommons.org/licenses/by/4.0/).

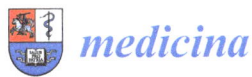

Article

The Association of Obstructive Sleep Apnea Syndrome and Accident Risk in Heavy Equipment Operators

Hakan Celikhisar [1,*] and Gulay Dasdemir Ilkhan [2]

1 Department of Chest Deseases, İzmir Metropolitan Municipality Hospital, İzmir 35110, Turkey
2 Department of Chest Diseases, Okmeydanı Training and Research Hospital, Istanbul 34384, Turkey; gulaydasdemir@gmail.com
* Correspondence: hcelikhisar@hotmail.com

Received: 25 June 2019; Accepted: 10 September 2019; Published: 17 September 2019

Abstract: *Background and Objectives*: Obstructive sleep apnea syndrome (OSAS) is the most frequent sleep disorder, characterized by the repeated collapse of the upper respiratory tract during sleep. In this study, we aimed to determine the prevalence of OSAS in heavy equipment operators and to determine the relationship between the work accidents that these operators were involved in and the OSAS symptoms and severity. In doing this, we aimed to emphasize the association of OSAS, which is a treatable disease, and these accidents, which cause loss of manpower, financial hampering, and even death. *Materials and Methods*: STOP BANG questionnaire was provided to 965 heavy equipment operators and polysomnography (PSG) was performed, in Izmir Esrefpasa Municipality Hospital, to the operators at high risk for OSAS. Demographic data, health status, and accidents of these operators were recorded. *Results*: All operators who participated in the study were male. The ages of the cases ranged from 35 to 58 and the mean age was 45.07 ± 5.54 years. The mean STOP BANG questionnaire results were 4.36 ± 3.82. In total, 142 operators were identified with high risk for OSAS and PSG could be performed on 110 of these 142 operators. According to the PSG results of the operators, 41 (37.3%) patients had normal findings, while 35 (31.8%) had mild, 20 (18.2%) had moderate, and 14 (12.7%) had severe OSAS. Among those 110 patients, 71 (64.5%) of the cases had no history of any accidents, 25 (22.8%) were almost involved in an accident due to sleepiness, and 14 (12.7%) were actually involved in an accident. There was a statistically significant relationship between the accident rate and OSAS severity (p: 0.009). *Conclusion*: Based on the data acquired in the present study, a positive correlation was determined between the accident statuses of drivers with OSAS severity. We want to attract attention to the necessity of evaluating the OSAS symptoms in professional heavy equipment operators during the certification period and at various intervals afterwards, and to carry out OSAS evaluations by PSG for those having a certain risk.

Keywords: polysomnography; heavy equipment operators; STOP BANG Questionnaire; Obstructive Sleep Apnea Syndrome

1. Introduction

Sleep is the temporary, partial, periodic, and reversible loss of the communication of the organism with the environment, which is an indispensable factor for a healthy life [1]. Obstructive sleep apnea syndrome (OSAS) is characterized by the repeated collapse of the upper respiratory tract during sleep, causing nocturnal hypoxemia and interrupted sleep [1]. It is the most frequent sleep disorder. OSAS prevalence has been determined as 3%–7% for males and 2%–5% for females all over the world [2].

The most common night symptom of OSAS is snoring, while the day symptom is excessive sleepiness [3,4]. The most important risk factors are indicated as male gender, advanced age, neck circumference, and obesity [5].

Various questionnaires are used for identifying risky groups and Berlin questionnaire is one of these arranged for community screenings. There are a total of 10 questions in three categories. Positive results in two or more categories indicate that the participant is carrying high risk [6]. STOP-BANG is another questionnaire defined to have high sensitivity to predict OSAS [7]. Polysomnography (PSG) is the gold standard in OSAS diagnosis and treatment management [5]. OSAS has been classified into three different classes according to apnea hypopnea index (AHI) as mild OSAS (AHI = 5–15), moderate OSAS (AHI = 15–30), and severe OSAS (AHI > 30) in accordance with the American Academy of Sleep Medicine Criteria [5]. Continuous positive air pressure (CPAP) is the standard treatment for OSAS [8,9].

Even though the nighttime symptoms of OSAS are generally ignored by the patient, its daytime symptoms are quite striking. Daytime excessive sleepiness may be so severe that it may affect work performance, prevent driving a vehicle carefully, and increase the accident risks [3]. For that reason, patients under high risk for OSAS should be diagnosed and treated. In this study, we aimed to determine the prevalence of OSAS in heavy equipment operators and to determine the relationship between the work accidents that these operators were involved in and the OSAS symptoms and severity. In this way, we aimed to emphasize the association of OSAS, which is a treatable disease, and these work accidents causing loss of manpower, financial hampering, and even death, which may be preventable.

2. Patients and Methods

The present study was planned as a prospective study at the Esrefpasa Municipality Hospital after the ethical approval was obtained from the Metropolitan Municipality (Number 54022451-050.05-04- from 1 February 2017). STOP BANG questionnaire was applied to 965 heavy equipment operators and PSG was performed in Izmir Esrefpasa Municipality Hospital to the operators at high risk for OSAS. The machines used by the operators include dumpers, hydraulic backhoes, crawled dozers, graders, wheeled front-end loaders, wheeled vibrating rollers, hydraulic breakers, drills, bucked wheel excavators, and backhoe loaders. Signed informed consent forms were obtained from all participants.

For the determination of STOP-BANG scores, snoring, daytime sleepiness (tiredness), observed apnea, high blood pressure (antihypertensive drug use), body mass index (positive if BMI > 35), age (positive if > 50 years), neck circumference (positive if > 40 cm.), and gender (male gender positive) were recorded. If participants chose the answer 'yes' for 3 of 8 questions; they were accepted as having high risk for OSAS.

Between February 2017 and March 2019, all of the operators examined in our hospital were male. Demographic characteristics such as age, weight, height, body mass index, neck circumference, waist/hip ratio, alcohol and cigarette smoking, and medical history were recorded. At the same time, the municipal official records of the accidents were questioned and recorded.

All patients included in our study were monitored all night by a trained sleep technician using a PSG device at our sleep center. At least 6 h of PSG recordings were acquired. Sleep staging and respiratory- and movement-scoring were done according to the American Academy of Sleep Medicine manual (version 2.0) by a sleep technician [10]. Apnea hypopnea index (AHI) was defined as the number of apneas and hypopneas per hour of sleep. Apnea was defined as the drop of airflow $\geq 90\%$ of baseline for at least 10 s and hypopnea as a decrease in airflow of at least 30% for at least 10 s with oxygen desaturation of more than 4% from baseline. The severity of OSA was determined by the AHI as mild if AHI is between 5 and 15, as moderate if AHI is between 15 and 30, and severe if AHI is greater than 30.

3. Statistical Analyses

IBM SPSS Statistics v. 22 (IBM Corp., Armonk, NY, USA) software was used for statistical analyses. Shapiro–Wilks test was used for evaluating the accordance of the parameters with normal distribution. In addition to descriptive statistical methods (mean, standard deviation, frequency), one-way ANOVA test was performed for the comparison of quantitative data, as well as Tukey HDS test and Tamhane's T2 test for the intergroup comparison of parameters with normal distribution and the determination of the group that causes the difference. Kruskal–Wallis test was used for carrying out intergroup comparisons of parameters without normal distribution. Whereas Chi Square test and Fisher–Freeman–Halton tests were performed for comparing qualitative data. Regression analysis was performed to determine the factors affecting the accident risk. Level of significance was evaluated as $p < 0.05$.

4. Results

The study was carried out between February 2017 and March 2019. In total, 142 operators were identified with high risk for OSAS and PSG could be performed on 110 of these 142 operators. All operators were male and their ages ranged from 35 to 58 years. The mean age of the operators was 45.07 ± 5.54 years. According to the PSG results of the study, 41 (37.3%) of the operators had normal findings, 35 (31.8%) had mild, 20 (18.2%) had moderate, and 14 (12.7%) had severe OSAS. The distribution of the general characteristics of the operators who participated in the study is shown in Table 1.

Table 1. Distribution of general characteristics.

	Min-Max	Mean ± SD
Age	35–58	42.07 ± 5.54
BMI * (kg/m^2)	21.89–42.14	31.89 ± 3.67
Neck circumference (cm)	34–52	42.32 ± 2.65
Waist to Hip ratio	0.81–1.13	0.96 ± 0.04
STOP BANG score	0–8	3.47 ± 3.73
Number of cigarette packs smoked annually	1–44	18.65 ± 7.89
Smoking		
Never smoked	34	30.90%
Quit smoking	20	18.50%
Current smoker	56	50.60%
Alcohol		
Not drinking	81	73.50%
Drinking	29	26.50%

*: Body Mass Index.

Of the cases, 87 (79.1%) did not have an accident, while 18 (16.4%) almost had an accident, and 5 (4.5%) had an accident. While 41 (37.3%) of the patients had normal PSG results, 35 (31.8%) had mild, 20 (18.2%) had moderate, and 14 (12.7%) had severe OSAS. The distribution of OSAS classification and accident status is summarized in Table 2. There was a statistically significant relationship between the accident rate and OSAS severity (*p*: 0.009).

Table 2. Distribution of obstructive sleep apnea syndrome (OSAS) classification and accident status.

	Normal (n: 41)	Mild OSAS (n: 35)	Moderate OSAS (n: 20)	Severe OSAS (n: 14)
No accident history	41 (100%)	29 (82.8%)	13 (65.0%)	4 (28.5%)
Almost involved in an accident	0	6 (17.2%)	6 (30.0%)	6 (43.0%)
Involved in an accident	0	0	1 (5.0%)	4 (28.5%)

The present results indicate that there was a statistically significant difference between accident histories with regard to apnea prevalence (p: 0.009). Apnea prevalence in those who had not been involved in any accident (37.2%) was observed to be lower at a statistically significant level in comparison to those who were almost involved in an accident due to sleepiness (64.8%) and those who were involved in an accident (61%) (p_1: 0.019; p_2: 0.047, respectively). No statistically significant difference with regard to apnea prevalence was observed between those who were almost involved in an accident due to sleepiness and those who had been involved in an accident ($p > 0.05$). A statistically significant difference was observed between accident histories with regard to snoring + apnea prevalence (p: 0.004). The snoring + apnea prevalence in those who had not been involved in any accident (35.8%) was observed to be lower at a statistically significant level in comparison to those who were almost involved in an accident (63.1%) and those who had been involved in an accident (62%) (p_1: 0.011; p_2: 0.031, respectively).

Table 3 presents the assessment of age, BMI, neck circumference, waist–hip ratio, and Epworth score among the OSAS classification groups.

Table 3. Evaluation of age, BMI, neck circumference, waist-hip ratio and STOP BANG, smoking and alcohol use states among OSAS classification groups.

	OSAS * Classification				p
	Normal (n: 41)	Mild OSAS (n: 35)	Moderate OSAS (n: 20)	Severe OSAS (n: 14)	
	Mean ± SD	Mean ± SD	Mean ± SD	Mean ± SD	
Age (years)	42.31 ± 5.8	41.39 ± 5.62	42.32 ± 6.08	42.34 ± 4.89	0.866
BMI ** (kg/m^2)	28.79 ± 2.7	30.98 ± 4.56	31.98 ± 3.31	34.01 ± 2.89	0.001 *
Neck circumference (cm)	40.99 ± 2.2	40.51 ± 3.22	41.45 ± 2.54	44.78 ± 2.1	0.001 *
Waist–Hip ratio	0.94 ± 0.04	0.94 ± 0.06	0.97 ± 0.04	0.98 ± 0.65	0.002 *
STOP BANG score	3.91 ± 2.4	4.69 ± 3.69	4.89 ± 4.59	4.37 ± 3.89	0.952
Epworth score	4.11 ± 2.09	4.31 ± 2.21	4.71 ± 2.21	4.89 ± 2.04	0.012

*: Obstructive sleep apnea syndrome, **: Body mass index.

According to the results of the present study, there was a statistically significant difference between the OSAS groups determined by PSG, regarding the BMI values and neck circumference (p: 0.001). The patients without OSAS had statistically significantly lower BMI values than those with moderate and severe OSAS (p_1: 0.032; p_2: 0.000, respectively). The BMI values of those with severe OSAS were determined to be higher at a statistically significant level in comparison with the BMI values of those with mild or moderate OSAS (p_1: 0.004; p_2: 0.017, respectively). The neck circumference values of those without OSAS were determined to be lower at a statistically significant level in comparison with that of the patients with moderate or severe OSAS (p_1: 0.019; p_2: 0.001, respectively). Neck circumference values of those with severe OSAS were determined to be higher at a statistically significant level in comparison with the mild OSAS group (p: 0.001). The waist–hip ratio of individuals with mild OSAS was determined to be lower at a statistically significant level in comparison with the waist–hip ratio of individuals with moderate or severe OSAS (p_1: 0.046; p_2: 0.004, respectively). Epworth score of the severe OSAS group was significantly higher than that of the healthy cases (p: 0.001).

There was a statistically significant difference between the OSAS groups with regard to accident status (p: 0.001;). The ratio of being almost involved in an accident due to sleepiness (0%) for drivers without OSAS was determined to be lower at a statistically significant level in comparison to drivers with mild (15.4%), moderate (28.6%), or severe (39.6%) OSAS (p_1: 0.026; p_2: 0.001; p_3: 0.001, respectively). The ratio of being involved in an accident for drivers with severe OSAS (34%) was determined to be higher at a statistically significant level in comparison to those of drivers with mild (0%) or moderate (5.7%) OSAS (p:0.001). No statistically significant difference could be determined between the drivers with mild and moderate OSAS with regard to the ratios of being involved in an accident ($p > 0.05$).

In Table 4, the results of regression analysis performed to determine the factors increasing accident risk are summarized. Regarding these findings, only AHI had significant effects on accident risk.

Table 4. Regression analysis performed to determine the factors increasing accident risk.

	t	p
BMI	−1.886	0.071
AHI	7.960	0.001
Epworth score	1.572	0.118
Waist/hip ratio	−0.291	0.772
Neck	1.107	0.270
STOP BANG score	−1.486	0.112

5. Discussion

Daytime sleepiness and loss of concentration is a common cause of accidents [11]. Short-term and poor quality sleep causes excessive daytime sleepiness, which increases the risk of accidents. Sleep disturbances such as obstructive sleep apnea syndrome are common causes of excessive sleepiness. In this study, in heavy equipment operators we determined a significant increase in accident risk with an increase in OSAS severity and in a regression analysis, there was a strong relationship between the AHI score and accident risk.

The studies on this subject are generally performed on long-distance drivers or taxi drivers, and the number of studies with the heavy equipment operators is limited. The majority of these studies are survey-oriented and the results obtained from the surveys are based on subjective data. Various surveys conducted with truck drivers showed a positive correlation between daytime excessive sleepiness and accidents [12–14]. In our study, we found that daytime sleepiness in heavy equipment operators was not a significant risk factor for accidents. However, this result may be related to the fact that the work was planned specifically for the heavy equipment operators and the maximum speed of the machines they were driving was limited at a speed of 20 km/h. However, in the case of heavy equipment operators, a distraction may cause serious accidents that can result in loss of life and property [15].

According to the results of STOP BANG survey, operators who were found to be at high risk for OSAS were evaluated with the results of PSG, performed in our sleep laboratory. Our study is one of the studies with a large sample group, which was performed with the participation of professional operators and evaluated the relationship between the accidents and PSG results. On the one hand, working with objective data will give more accurate results, on the other hand, the difficulty of doing PSG for each participant may be the obvious reason for not giving up surveys. Subjective symptoms such as snoring and apnea, which are questioned in terms of OSAS, are the symptoms they cannot detect on their own. On the other hand, financial anxiety may result in bias and the surveys may not reflect the realities. Results with similar concerns may be deceptive during job applications or health checks. Therefore, OSAS symptom questioning alone may be inadequate, and delays in diagnosis and treatment of OSAS cases may cause severe issues for the patients as well as the society due to the accidents [16,17]. With this fact, in some parts of the European Union countries, driver's licenses are not given to OSAS patients because they do not have healthy driver qualifications [18,19].

The STOP BANG questionnaire was used to determine daytime sleepiness. In our study, the STOP BANG questionnaire score was below three in the majority of patients, including those describing daytime sleepiness (EDS). Regarding this data, the STOP BANG questionnaire completed by the operators may be suggested as inadequate and unsuitable for determining the EDS. We also did not determine an association between STOP BANG score and accident risk in regression analysis. On the other hand, the work and material concerns of our patients may make the questionnaire-based survey results illusory.

When compared to normal healthy individuals, accidents with OSAS operators were reported to be seen seven times higher [20,21]. As the apnea hypopnea index (AHI) increased in the study of Young et al., the risk of accident was found to be increased, in accordance with our study [22]. In another study by Teran-Santos et al., a significant relationship was found between the risk of accident and presence of OSAS. According to the results of the same study, when the operators with OSAS were evaluated with the increase in severity of the disease, the risk of accidents also increased, in parallel with our study. Accident rates in our study were determined as 28.5% in severe OSAS, 5.0% in moderate OSAS, and 0% in mild OSAS patients. Statistically, these rates show a positive correlation between the severity of OSAS and accident frequency. On the other hand, according to the results of STOP BANG survey, PSG was performed on a high-risk group and some of them did not have OSAS. No accident history was found in healthy group. Regarding the demographic data in our study; body mass index (BMI), neck circumference, and waist–hip ratio did not show any association with the accident risk. However, in the study of Amra et al., increased neck circumference was determined as a factor increasing the risk of accident [13].

In the light of all these data, it seems that the questioning of OSAS symptoms alone will not be enough to predict the risk of accidents. However, there are many studies demonstrating the relationship between the severity of OSAS and accident risk. Regarding the increased morbidity and mortality due to the accidents, it is a necessity to inquire about the OSAS symptoms in the professional drivers, such as heavy equipment operators, during the certification phase and to perform polysomnography on the drivers with high risk. It is concluded that in order to prevent the morbidity and mortalities, in the groups involved in the field of occupational risk, routine PSG studies may be required. For this purpose, it is necessary to question the number of sleep centers and to determine the OSAS symptoms periodically during the certification and after, and to increase the screening.

There are some limitations of this study that should be mentioned. The STOP BANG questionnaire is based on the patient responses, and this may carry some bias that the vehicle operators may not respond correctly; since they may be afraid of losing their job. Second, this is the report of single center results and larger, prospective studies investigating the treatment responses in this group of patients are warranted.

6. Conclusions

We want to attract attention to the necessity of evaluating the OSAS symptoms of professional heavy equipment operators during the certification period and at various intervals afterwards and to carry out OSAS evaluations by PSG for those with a certain risk.

Author Contributions: Conceptualization, H.C.; Methodology, G.D.I.; Software, H.C.; Validation, G.D.I.; Formal Analysis, G.D.I.; Investigation, H.C.; Resources, H.C.; Data Curation, G.D.I.; Writing—Original Draft Preparation G.D.I.; Writing—Review & Editing, H.C.; Visualization, G.D.I.; Supervision, G.D.I.; Project Administration, H.C.

Funding: This research received no external funding.

Conflicts of Interest: The authors declare no conflict of interest.

References

1. Sateia, M.J. International classification of sleep disorders. *Chest* **2014**, *146*, 1387–1394. [CrossRef] [PubMed]
2. Punjabi, N.M. The epidemiology of adult obstructive sleep apnea. *Proc. Am. Thorac. Soc.* **2008**, *5*, 136–143. [CrossRef] [PubMed]
3. Kacem, I.; Kalboussi, H.; Ben, H.S.; Maoua, M.; El, S.G.; Laayouni, M.; Abdelghani, A.; Boughattas, W.; Brahem, A.; Debbabi, F.; et al. Quality of life in adult patient (Tunisian) with severe OSA. *Rev. Pneumol. Clin.* **2017**, *73*, 163–171. [CrossRef] [PubMed]
4. Hongyo, K.; Ito, N.; Yamamoto, K.; Yasunobe, Y.; Takeda, M.; Oguro, R.; Takami, Y.; Takeya, Y.; Sugimoto, K.; Rakugi, H. Factors associated with the severity of obstructive sleep apnea in older adults. *Geriatr. Gerontol. Int.* **2017**, *17*, 614–621. [CrossRef] [PubMed]
5. Foldvary-Schaefer, N.R.; Waters, T.E. Sleep-disordered breathing. Continuum (Minneap Minn). *Sleep Disord. Breath.* **2017**, *23*, 1093–1116.
6. Ng, S.S.; Tam, W.; Chan, T.O.; To, K.W.; Ngai, J.; Chan, K.K.P.; Yip, W.H.; Lo, R.L.; Yiu, K.; Ko, F.W.; et al. Use of Berlin questionnaire in comparison to polysomnography and home sleep study in patients with obstructive sleep apnea. *Respir. Res.* **2019**, *20*, 40. [CrossRef] [PubMed]
7. Saldías Peñafiel, F.; Gassmann Poniachik, J.; Canelo López, A.; Uribe Monasterio, J.; Díaz Patiño, O. Accuracy of sleep questionnaires for obstructive sleep apnea syndrome screening. *Rev. Med. Chil.* **2018**, *146*, 1123–1134. [CrossRef] [PubMed]
8. Xanthopoulos, M.S.; Kim, J.Y.; Blechner, M.; Chang, M.-Y.; Menello, M.K.; Brown, C.; Matthews, E.; Weaver, T.E.; Shults, J.; Marcus, C.L. Self-efficacy and short-term adherence to continuous positive airway pressure treatment in children. *Sleep* **2017**, *40*, zsx096. [CrossRef] [PubMed]
9. Freedman, N. Treatment of obstructive sleep apnea: Choosing the best positive airway pressure device. *Sleep Med. Clin.* **2017**, *12*, 529–542. [CrossRef]
10. Garbarino, S.; Scoditti, E.; Lanteri, P.; Conte, L.; Magnavita, N.; Toraldo, D.M. Obstructive sleep apnea with or without excessive daytime sleepiness: Clinical and experimental data-driven phenotyping. *Front. Neurol.* **2018**, *9*, 505. [CrossRef] [PubMed]
11. Fantus, R.J. Asleep at the wheel: Obstructive sleep apnea. *Bull. Am. Coll. Surg.* **2017**, *102*, 57–58. [PubMed]
12. Amra, B.; Dorali, R.; Mortazavi, S.; Golshan, M.; Farajzadegan, Z.; Fietze, I.; Penzel, T. Sleep & breathing Sleep apnea symptoms and accident risk factors in Persian commercial vehicle drivers = Schlaf & Atmung. *Sleep Breath.* **2012**, *16*, 187–191. [PubMed]
13. Al-Abri, M.A.; Al-Adawi, S.; Al-Abri, I.; Al-Abri, F.; Dorvlo, A.; Wesonga, R.; Jaju, S. Daytime sleepiness among young adult Omani car drivers. *Sultan Qaboos Univ. Med. J.* **2018**, *18*, e143. [CrossRef]
14. Teran-Santos, J.; Jimenez-Gomez, A.; Cordero-Guevara, J.; the Cooperative Group Burgos–Santander. The association between sleep apnea and the risk of traffic accidents. *N. Engl. J. Med.* **1999**, *340*, 847–851. [CrossRef] [PubMed]
15. Lemos, L.C.; Marqueze, E.C.; Sachi, F.; Lorenzi-Filho, G.; Moreno, C.R.d.C.M. Obstructive sleep apnea syndrome in truck drivers. *J. Bras. Pneumol.* **2009**, *35*, 500–506. [CrossRef] [PubMed]
16. Garbarino, S.; Durando, P.; Guglielmi, O.; Dini, G.; Bersi, F.; Fornarino, S.; Toletone, A.; Chiorri, C.; Magnavita, N. Sleep apnea, sleep debt and daytime sleepiness are independently associated with road accidents. A cross-sectional study on truck drivers. *PLoS ONE* **2016**, *11*, e0166262. [CrossRef]
17. Guglielmi, O.; Magnavita, N.; Garbarino, S. Sleep quality, obstructive sleep apnea, and psychological distress in truck drivers: A cross-sectional study. *Soc. Psychiatry Psychiatr. Epidemiol.* **2018**, *53*, 531–536. [CrossRef]
18. Garbarino, S.; Guglielmi, O.; Campus, C.; Mascialino, B.; Pizzorni, D.; Nobili, L.; LuigiMancardi, G.; Ferini-Stramb, L. Screening, diagnosis, and management of obstructive sleep apnea in dangerous-goods truck drivers: To be aware or not? *Sleep Med.* **2016**, *25*, 98–104. [CrossRef]
19. Vennelle, M.; Engleman, H.M.; Douglas, N.J. Sleepiness and sleep-related accidents in commercial bus drivers. *Sleep Breath.* **2010**, *14*, 39–42. [CrossRef]
20. George, C.J.T. Sleep·5: Driving and automobile crashes in patients with obstructive sleep apnoea/hypopnoea syndrome. *Thorax* **2004**, *59*, 804–807. [CrossRef]

21. Young, T.; Blustein, J.; Finn, L.; Palta, M. Sleep-disordered breathing and motor vehicle accidents in a population-based sample of employed adults. *Sleep* **1997**, *20*, 608–613. [CrossRef] [PubMed]
22. Terán Santos, J.; Moreno, G.; Rodenstein, D.O. Sleep medicine and transport workers. Medico-social aspects with special reference to sleep apnea syndrome. *Arch. Bronconeumol.* **2010**, *46*, 143–147. [CrossRef] [PubMed]

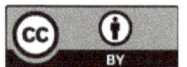

© 2019 by the authors. Licensee MDPI, Basel, Switzerland. This article is an open access article distributed under the terms and conditions of the Creative Commons Attribution (CC BY) license (http://creativecommons.org/licenses/by/4.0/).

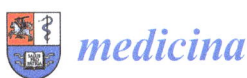

Article

Particularities of Older Patients with Obstructive Sleep Apnea and Heart Failure with Mid-Range Ejection Fraction

Carmen Loredana Ardelean [1,*], Sorin Pescariu [2], Daniel Florin Lighezan [2], Roxana Pleava [1,*], Sorin Ursoniu [3], Valentin Nadasan [4] and Stefan Mihaicuta [5]

1. University of Medicine and Pharmacy, Dr Victor Babes, Eftimie Murgu Square 2, 300041 Timisoara, Romania
2. Cardiology Department, University of Medicine and Pharmacy, Dr Victor Babes, Eftimie Murgu Square 2, 300041 Timisoara, Romania
3. Department of Public Health and Health Management, University of Medicine and Pharmacy, Dr Victor Babes, Eftimie Murgu Square 2, 300041 Timisoara, Romania
4. Department of Hygiene and Environmental Health, University of Medicine and Pharmacy, Sciences and Technology of Targu Mures, Gheorghe Marinescu 38, 540139 Targu Mures, Romania
5. Pneumology Department, University of Medicine and Pharmacy, Dr Victor Babes, Eftimie Murgu Square 2, 300041 Timisoara, Romania
* Correspondence: carmenardelean79@yahoo.com (C.L.A.); roxana.pleava@gmail.com (R.P.); Tel.: +00-407-2410-5175 (C.L.A.); +407-6555-8929 (R.P.)

Received: 22 June 2019; Accepted: 5 August 2019; Published: 7 August 2019

Abstract: *Background and objectives*: Obstructive sleep apnea syndrome (OSAS) and heart failure (HF) are increasing in prevalence with a greater impact on the health system. The aim of this study was to assess the particularities of patients with OSAS and HF, focusing on the new class of HF with mid-range ejection fraction (HFmrEF, EF = 40%–49%), and comparing it with reduced EF (HFrEF, EF < 40%) and preserved EF (HFpEF, EF ≥ 50%). *Materials and Methods*: A total of 143 patients with OSAS and HF were evaluated in three sleep labs of "Victor Babes" Hospital and Cardiovascular Institute, Timisoara, Western Romania. We collected socio-demographic data, anthropometric sleep-related measurements, symptoms through sleep questionnaires and comorbidity-related data. We performed blood tests, cardio-respiratory polygraphy and echocardiographic measurements. Patients were divided into three groups depending on ejection fraction. *Results*: Patients with HFmrEF were older ($p = 0.0358$), with higher values of the highest systolic blood pressure (mmHg) ($p = 0.0016$), higher serum creatinine ($p = 0.0013$), a lower glomerular filtration rate ($p = 0.0003$), higher glycemic levels ($p = 0.008$) and a larger left atrial diameter ($p = 0.0002$). Regarding comorbidities, data were presented as percentage, HFrEF vs. HFmrEF vs. HFpEF. Higher prevalence of diabetes mellitus (52.9 vs. 72.7 vs. 40.2, $p = 0.006$), chronic kidney disease (17.6 vs. 57.6 vs. 21.5, $p < 0.001$), tricuspid insufficiency (76.5 vs. 84.8 vs.59.1, $p = 0.018$) and aortic insufficiency (35.3 vs.42.4 vs. 20.4, $p = 0.038$) were observed in patients with HFmrEF, whereas chronic obstructive pulmonary disease(COPD) (52.9 vs. 24.2 vs.18.3, $p = 0.009$), coronary artery disease(CAD) (82.4 vs. 6.7 vs. 49.5, $p = 0.026$), myocardial infarction (35.3 vs. 24.2 vs. 5.4, $p < 0.001$) and impaired parietal heart kinetics (70.6 vs. 68.8 vs. 15.2, $p < 0.001$) were more prevalent in patients with HFrEF. *Conclusions*: Patients with OSAS and HF with mid-range EF may represent a new group with increased risk of developing life-long chronic kidney disease, diabetes mellitus, tricuspid and aortic insufficiency. COPD, myocardial infarction, impaired parietal kinetics and CAD are most prevalent comorbidities in HFrEF patients but they are closer in prevalence to HFmrEF than HFpEF.

Keywords: obstructive apnea; heart failure; risk factors; elderly; comorbidities

1. Introduction

In recent years, obstructive sleep apnea syndrome (OSAS) has increased in prevalence, occurring in up to 10% of healthy subjects, due to the greater frequency of obesity and the aging of the population. Consequently, this has had an increasingly important impact on the health system [1]. The prevalence of OSAS in subjects with cardiovascular disease, reported in earlier studies, was between 50% and 80% [2–4], and in half of subjects with heart failure (HF), it is associated with increased mortality [5] and worse prognosis [6].

OSAS is globally known as a major factor for the occurrence of cardiometabolic comorbidities due to intermittent hypoxia which leads to oxidative stress, endothelial dysfunction, increase of sympathetic activity and systemic inflammation [7]. Furthermore, activation of the sympathetic nervous system leads to activation of the renin-angiotensin-aldosterone system, which increases hydro-saline retention and thus the level of blood pressure [8]. However, hydro-saline retention due to heart failure can also play an important role in the pathogenesis of OSAS [9]. These data suggest that the relationship between HF and OSAS is not fully understood.

Large studies have demonstrated that OSAS prevalence is higher in patients with coronary artery disease (CAD), HF, resistant arterial hypertension associated with risk of stroke, and uncontrolled arrhythmias [10].

Patients with OSAS present a variety of symptoms that correlate with anthropometric measurements, smoking habits, sedentarism and association of comorbidities [1]. In recent years, new perspectives regarding clinical presentations of OSAS with description of different phenotypes and clusters have emerged [11–13].

Different structural or functional cardiac abnormalities can lead to occurrence of typical symptoms and signs of HF as defined by the European Society of Cardiology (ESC) guidelines, increased morbidity and mortality and higher costs for the health system [14]. HF is more common in elderly patients, especially those over 60 years [15].

The measurement of the left ventricle ejection fraction (LVEF) is used to define HF. Accordingly, HF is classified as HF with preserved LVEF, ≥50% (HFpEF) and HF with reduced LVEF, <40% (HFrEF). Recently, the latest guidelines on the diagnosis and management of heart failure published by the European Society of Cardiology proposed a new class of HF patients with LVEF = 40%–49% called HF with mid-range EF (HFmrEF), in order to better differentiate HF patients from the point of view of etiology, developing mechanisms and response to treatment strategy [16,17].

2. Materials and Methods

2.1. Study Subjects

We enrolled consecutive patients evaluated for OSAS at the "Victor Babes" Timisoara Hospital between 2014 and 2018 and for HF at the Timisoara Institute for Cardiovascular Diseases. Inclusion criteria were patients with age over 40 years, with a diagnosis of heart failure and OSAS who performed cardio-respiratory polygraphy, echocardiography and blood test evaluation. Patients with incomplete evaluation and those with no OSAS or with predominantly central sleep apnea (CSA) were excluded. This study was approved by the Ethical Committee of the University of Medicine and Pharmacy "Victor Babes" Timisoara as a subject for a PhD thesis (number 14728/15 NOV 2013). The clinics where the patient's evaluations were performed have an established agreement with the university through which all the data obtained from the patients may be used for research purposes. Informed consent was signed by all the patients.

Patients were initially evaluated through a standard datasheet with the following parameters: Age (years), gender (male/female), weight (kg) and height (cm), followed by measurement of body mass index (BMI = weight in kg/squared height in m), neck and abdominal circumference (cm), presence and duration of hypertension, maximum and current value of blood pressure, medication, reported apneas, snoring, sleepiness, Epworth Sleepiness Scale, SAS score (sleep apnea syndrome score), morning headache, restless sleep, nocturia, nocturnal awakenings, chronic obstructive pulmonary disease (COPD), diabetes, dyslipidemia, CAD, HF, arrhythmias, stroke, nasal septum deviation, polyposis, hypertrophic uvula and smoking status (pack × years). Since it is not routine practice in our cardio-respiratory unit, we did not collect data about physical activity.

For the sleep study we followed the European standards for diagnosis of OSAS [18].

Cardio-respiratory polygraphy recording was performed with Stardust Respironics and Porti. Several parameters were measured: The number of apnea (individually, central, obstructive and mixed) and hypopnea per hour of sleep and per night, the AHI (apnea-hypopnea index), the desaturation index, the mean saturation, the lowest saturation, and the longest desaturation period below 88% (seconds). Because we did not perform full night assisted polysomnography, data about sleep duration and duration of the lowest desaturation were not recorded. Approximately one-third of the patients enrolled in this study used CPAP (continuous positive airway pressure) due to the non-reimbursement of the cost of this therapy. Therefore, data related to the use of CPAP have not been included in this study.

The cardio-respiratory polygraphy recording was performed and scored manually as stated by American Academy of Sleep Medicine standards and European Sleep Research Society recommendations [19].

Laboratory tests were performed in Romanian Accreditation Association-RENAR certified medical laboratories, as follows: ESR (erythrocyte sedimentation rate) (mm/h), glucose (mg/dL), uric acid (mg/dL), creatinine (mg/dL), erythrocyte count (×10^6/µL), hemoglobin (g/dL), sodium (mmol/L), potassium (mmol/L) and lipid profile (total cholesterol, LDL (low-density lipoprotein)-cholesterol, HDL (high-density lipoprotein)-cholesterol, triglycerides, mg/dl). Glomerular filtration rate, (GFR, mL/min/1.73 m^2) was calculated for each patient, using CKD-EPI (Chronic Kidney Disease Epidemiology Collaboration) formula [20]. Blood samples were collected early in the morning after fasting, and within 1–2 days of informed consent if signing took place at a different time of day.

Cardiological evaluation was performed, for all patients, at the Institute of Cardiovascular Diseases in Timisoara, using the same diagnostic algorithm and equipment. We used the modified Simpson's rule for echocardiographic measurement of EF [21], and HF was classified depending on the LVEF, HF with preserved ejection fraction, LVEF ≥ 50% (HFpEF); HF with reduced ejection fraction, LVEF < 40% (HFrEF); and HF with mid-range ejection fraction, LVEF = 40%–49% (HFmrEF). We also recorded end-diastolic volume (mL), end-systolic volume (mL), left atrium surface (cm^2), left atrium diameter (cm), right ventricle diameter (cm), mitral E and A wave (m/s), E/A ratio, pulmonary artery pression (mm Hg) and percentage of patients with impaired parietal heart kinetics. Although, the assessment of the left ventricular internal dimension, left ventricular posterior wall, interventricular septum thickness is performed in current practice and provides valuable information about the HF etiology, in this study they were not recorded because we enrolled patients with heart failure, regardless of the underlying cardiac disease. We studied patients regarding LVEF only, as the main cardiac marker.

The morphological aspect, area (cm), degree of regurgitation and stenoses and transvalvular pressure gradients were determined for the mitral, aortic, tricuspid and pulmonary valves [22].

2.2. Statistical Analysis

Data are presented as proportions, medians and interquartile range (IQR) for variables with a skewed distribution. The differences in the characteristics of the subjects were evaluated after being divided into three groups, depending on the EF (EF < 40%, EF = 40%–49%, EF ≥ 50%). We used the chi-squared test (two degrees of freedom) for comparison of categorical data between groups of patients. Continuous data were tested for normality using the Kolmogorov–Smirnov test. Data with non-normal distributions were compared using the Kruskal–Wallis test. The p values for all hypothesis tests were two-sided, and the p value was set to the statistical significance threshold of <0.005. All data analyses were performed with Stata 15.1 (Statacorp, TX, USA).

3. Results

A total of 143 patients with OSAS and HF were evaluated in three sleep labs of Timisoara "Victor Babes" Hospital, Western Romania.

3.1. Socio-Demographic and Anthropometric Data

Patients were divided into three groups depending on EF, with the following characteristics, presented as median and interquartile range: 17 patients (11.88%) with HFrEF, of which 15 male (88%), age 61 (56–69) years, BMI 35 (31–36) kg/m^2, neck circumference 44 (39–46) cm, abdominal circumference 120 (114–128) cm; 33 patients (23.07%) with HFmrEF, of which 22 male (67%), age 64.5 (57.5–71) years, BMI 36 (31.5–41.5) kg/m^2, neck circumference 45 (42–46) cm, abdominal circumference 120 (114–130) cm; 93 patients (65.93%) with HFpEF, of which 62 male (67%), BMI 35 (31–41) kg/m^2, neck circumference 44 (41–46) cm, abdominal circumference 122 (115–130) cm (Table 1).

Table 1. Socio-demographic and anthropometric data.

General Data	EF < 40% (HFrEF) n = 17	EF = 40%–49% (HFmrEF) n = 33	EF ≥ 50% (HFpEF) n = 93	p-Value
Age (years)	61 (56–69)	64.5 (57.5–71)	61 (56–67)	0.0358
Male (no., %)	15 (88%)	22 (67%)	62 (67%)	0.187
BMI (kg/m^2)	35 (31–36)	36 (31.5–41.5)	35 (31–41)	0.415
Neck circumference (cm)	44 (39–46)	45 (42–46)	44 (41–46)	0.6573
Abdominal circumference (cm)	120 (114–128)	120 (114–130)	122 (115–130)	0.8569

Data are presented as proportions, medians and interquartile range (IQR). EF, ejection fraction; HFrEF, heart failure with reduced ejection fraction; HFmrEF, heart failure with mid-range EF; HFpEF, heart failure with preserved EF; BMI, body mass index.

Patients from the HFmrEF group were significantly older. More males were found in the HFrEF group. There were no differences in terms of BMI, neck and abdominal circumference (Table 1).

3.2. Sleep Study and Blood Pressure Data

There were no differences between groups of patients regarding blood pressure (BP) measurement and sleep study, systolic and diastolic BP at visit, AHI, type of apneas, desaturation index, medium and lowest desaturation, longest desaturation <88% and sleep questionnaire. Significant differences were observed in patients with HFmrEF regarding the highest systolic BP reported by the patients ($p = 0.016$) (Table 2).

Table 2. Blood pressure and sleep study.

Sleep/Blood Pressure Parameters	EF < 40% (HFrEF) n = 17	EF = 40%–49% (HFmrEF) n = 33	EF ≥ 50% (HFpEF) n = 93	p-Value
Highest Systolic BP (mmHg)	161 (161–179)	202 (177.5–220)	191 (170–210)	**0.0016**
Highest Diastolic BP (mmHg)	90 (80–100)	100 (90–110)	100 (90–110)	0.1472
Duration of hypertension (years)	12 (7–20)	10 (8–14.5)	10 (5–15)	0.3899
AHI (events/h)	42 (24–53)	38 (24–48.5)	44 (27–62)	0.1633
Central apneas	1 (0.4–9.5)	1.25 (0.25–4.66)	1.7 (0.3–5.4)	0.8947
Obstructive apneas	13.2 (8.9–21.3)	14.55 (7.2–23.8)	19.2 (12–38.2)	0.0704
Mixed apneas	2 (0.9–6)	1.75 (0.45–3.2)	2.1 (0.7–6.1)	0.3153
Desaturation index	24 (14.5–51)	30.5 (13.4–46.4)	39.5 (19–53)	0.1856
Medium SpO2 (%)	93 (90–94)	92.5 (91–94)	92 (89–93)	0.1403
Lowest SpO2 (%)	78 (76–83)	76 (66–83)	77 (62–83)	0.6183
Longest duration SpO2 <88% (sec)	50 (21–115)	61 (27–110.5)	83 (30–139)	0.3311
Epworth Sleepiness Scale	13 (12–17)	12 (9–15)	13 (10–18)	0.0819
SAS score	4.9 (4.5–5.4)	4.3 (4.1–4.85)	4.8 (4.1–5.3)	0.0857

Data are presented as medians and interquartile range (IQR). BP, blood pressure; AHI, apnea-hypopnea index; SpO2, oxygen saturation; SAS score, sleep apneas syndrome score.

3.3. Blood Tests

Routine blood tests revealed significant statistical difference in HFmrEF patients regarding level of glucose ($p = 0.0081$), creatinine ($p = 0.0013$) and GFR ($p = 0.0003$) (Table 3). There were no differences for ESR, uric acid, erythrocytes, hemoglobin, Na, K, total cholesterol, LDL and HDL cholesterol, or triglycerides.

Table 3. Blood tests.

Blood Tests	EF < 40% (HFrEF) $n = 17$	EF = 40%–49% (HFmrEF) $n = 33$	EF ≥ 50% (HFpEF) $n = 93$	p-Value
ESR (mm/h)	10.5 (8–25)	15 (8–32)	12 (6–25)	0.4202
Glucose (mg/dL)	122.5 (104–130.5)	126 (107–180.5)	108.5 (94–127)	**0.0081**
Uric acid (mg/dL)	7 (4.9–8.3)	6.6 (5.2–8.1)	5.9 (5–6.9)	0.2547
Creatinine (mg/dL)	1.15 (0.98–1.3)	1.33 (1.13–1.6)	1.075 (0.9–1.33)	**0.0013**
GFR (mL/min/1.73 m^2)	61.8 (58.9–78)	48.8 (38.7–61)	65.7 (51.3–82.3)	**0.0003**
Erythrocytes(*10^6/μL)	4.73 (4.42–5.06)	4.80 (4.45–5.13)	4.77 (4.43–5.12)	0.8399
Hemoglobin (g/dL)	14.1 (12–15.9)	14 (12.3–15.1)	14.5 (13.2–15.45)	0.3972
Na+ (mmol/L)	140 (138.5–142)	141 (139–144)	141 (139–142)	0.5287
K+ (mmol/L)	4.13 (4–4.65)	4.35 (3.9–4.)	4.2 (4–4.6)	0.8157
Cholesterol (mg/dL)	166 (143–182.5)	163 (130–195)	164 (135–205)	0.9128
LDL cholesterol (mg/dL)	123 (87–132)	94.5 (84–117)	98 (69–132)	0.9003
HDL cholesterol (mg/dL)	45 (36–48)	45 (32–54)	43 (37–52)	0.7776
Triglycerides (mg/dL)	128.5 (90–166)	96 (82–151)	125 (92–193)	0.3465

Data are presented as medians and interquartile range (IQR). ESR, erythrocyte sedimentation rate; GFR, glomerular Filtration Rate; LDL, low-density lipoprotein; HDL, high-density lipoprotein.

3.4. Echocardiographic Measurements

Regarding echocardiographic measurements, statistically significant differences were found for end-diastolic and end-systolic volumes, ejection fraction, and left atrial diameter. LA (left atrium) diameter was higher in patients with HFmrEF ($p = 0.0002$), similar to other publications (Table 4)

Table 4. Echocardiographic measurements.

Echocardiography Parameters	EF < 40% (HFrEF) $n = 17$	EF = 40%–49% (HFmrEF) $n = 33$	EF ≥ 50% (HFpEF) $n = 93$	p-Value
End–diastolic volume (ml)	185 (140–220)	118 (94–155)	130 (110–147.5)	**0.0027**
End–systolic volume (ml)	123.5 (90–154)	64.9 (53–84.5)	60 (48.5–65.5)	**0.0001**
EF (%)	31.58 (30–35.71)	44.87 (43.37–46.13)	55 (50.98–59)	**0.0001**
LA surface (cm^2)	27 (21–32)	28 (24.5–31)	25 (23–29)	0.4666
LA diameter (cm)	4.7 (4.6–5)	4.95 (4.5–5.3)	4.3 (3.9–4.64)	**0.0002**
RV diameter (cm)	3.24 (2.5–3.6)	2.9 (2.6–3.25)	2.8 (2.5–3.14)	0.2684
Mitral E wave (m/s)	0.74 (0.63–1)	0.76 (0.58–1.07)	0.73 (0.55–0.9)	0.298
Mitral A wave (m/s)	0.70 (0.5–1.07)	0.8 (0.6–1)	0.7 (0.6–0.9)	0.6517
E/A ratio	0.86 (0.74–1.65)	0.79 (0.64–1.4)	0.87 (0.73–1.3)	0.6883
PAP (mmHg)	47.5 (25–63.3)	45 (34.5–50)	36 (25.5–45.5)	0.1303

Data are presented as medians and interquartile range (IQR). LA, Left atrium; RV, right ventricle; PAP, pulmonary artery pressure.

3.5. Comorbidities

Regarding comorbidities, data were presented as proportions, HFrEF vs. HFmrEF vs. HFpEF. We observed that the group with HFmrEF has significantly more cases of diabetes mellitus (52.9 vs. 72.7 vs. 40.2 $p = 0.006$), chronic kidney disease (17.6 vs. 57.6 vs. 21.5, $p < 0.001$), valvular disease, tricuspid insufficiency (76.5 vs. 84.8 vs. 59.1, $p = 0.018$) and aortic insufficiency (35.3 vs. 42.4 vs. 20.4, $p = 0.038$). The group with HFrEF had more cases of COPD (52.9 vs. 24.2 vs. 18.3, $p = 0.009$), myocardial infarction (35.3 vs. 24.2. vs 5.4, $p < 0.001$), CAD (82.4 vs. 66.7 vs. 49.5, $p = 0.026$) and impaired heart parietal kinetics (70.6 vs. 68.8 vs. 15.2, $p < 0.001$). The presence of myocardial infarction,

CAD and impaired heart parietal kinetics were much lower in HFpEF patients compared with HFmrEF and HFrEF (Table 5).

Table 5. Comorbidities.

Comorbidities %	EF < 40% (HFrEF) $n = 17$	EF = 40%–49% (HFmrEF) $n = 33$	EF ≥ 50% (HFpEF) $n = 93$	p-Value
Hypertension	100	97	95.7	0.670
Smoking	35.3	15.2	36.6	0.070
COPD	52.9	24.2	18.3	**0.009**
Diabetes mellitus	52.9	72.7	40.2	**0.006**
Dyslipidemia	76.5	66.7	66.7	0.719
Atrial fibrillation	58.8	57.6	37.6	0.065
Stroke	5.9	6.1	12.9	0.781
Myocardial infarction	35.3	24.2	5.4	**<0.001**
CAD	82.4	66.7	49.5	**0.026**
CKD	17.6	57.6	21.5	**<0.001**
Mitral insufficiency	94.1	90.9	77.4	0.088
Tricuspid insufficiency	76.5	84.8	59.1	**0.018**
Aortic insufficiency	35.3	42.4	20.4	**0.038**
Pulmonary insufficiency	17.65	15.63	12.9	0.840
PAH	47.1	39.4	25.8	0.298
Pulmonary thromboembolism	5.9	3.0	5.4	0.863
Impaired parietal heart kinetics	70.6	68.8	15.2	**<0.001**

COPD, chronic obstructive pulmonary disease; CAD, coronary artery disease; CDK, chronic kidney disease; PAH, pulmonary arterial hypertension.

4. Discussion

In our population, 23.07 % of the patients had HFmrEF, higher than reports from recent studies where the percentage of the HFmrEF category is between 13% and 17% [23–26].

Men are more likely to have OSAS in patients with HF. Moreover, men have a higher incidence of HF in patients with OSAS [27]. In our study, patients with HFmrEF were older, with no significant differences regarding gender or neck and abdominal circumferences.

It is well known that obesity is an important risk factor for heart failure, and this association leads to multiple complications. In addition, obesity seems to be more prevalent in HF patients with preserved ejection fraction; this may occur due to poor echocardiographic images and error in LVEF measurement [28]. In our study, we included only patients with OSAS, and patients with HFmrEF were in stage 2 of obesity, with higher BMIs, but differences were not statistically significant. Central sleep apnea (CSA) is particularly noted in patients with HFrEF, and decompensated HF has been recognized as a risk factor for CSA [29].

Some studies have demonstrated that patients with heart failure and OSAS are less symptomatic, regardless of AHI, and Epworth Sleepiness Scale does not correlate with AHI [30]. Questionnaires do not accurately predict OSAS in patients with cardio-vascular disease (CVD) [31]. Epworth Sleepiness Scale and SAS score can be beneficial in predicting OSAS, but in our groups of patients, although the values are high, differences between groups are insignificant [32].

In our group, all the patients have severe OSAS, regardless of EF. Patients with severe, untreated OSAS have a higher risk of fatal cardiovascular events, some studies show [33].

Our patients with HFmrEF have higher blood glucose, serum creatinine and decreased glomerular filtration rate.

Nielson demonstrated in a large study that patients with elevated blood glucose levels but without confirmed diabetes have an increased risk of developing HF. Therefore, these patients should be carefully monitored in order to prevent the onset of HF [34].

Many studies demonstrated that even mild impaired renal function, with transitory elevated level of serum creatinine, represents an important predictor for worsening of heart failure.

The pathophysiology remains unclear, but venous congestion and intrabdominal pressure serve as a challenge for the development of new therapeutic approaches [35,36]. OSAS severity was correlated with elevated serum creatinine [37], while CKD stage 3 is considered a significant predictor of CSA, as was demonstrated by Fleischmann et al. [38].

In this study, lipid profile is not different as in a cohort with all severities of disease where OSAS severity was independently correlated with cholesterol and triglycerides levels, probably because all our patients have severe OSAS [39].

Often, patients with HFpEF present only increased wall thickness of the LV or the size of LA, which makes it even more difficult to diagnose. In our study, LA diameter was higher in patients with HFmrEF ($p = 0.0002$), similar to other publications [40]. Moreover, the role of the left atrium in modulating LV function is well-known [41], and there are considerable amounts of data demonstrating that the size of the LA is directly proportional to the increased risk of cardiovascular events; this parameter is not used enough in clinical practice to determine the HF progression [42].

Wang et al. demonstrated in a recent meta-analysis that patients with moderate to severe tricuspid regurgitation (TR) have a higher risk of hospitalization for worsening HF and cardiac mortality. Patients with TR, regardless of severity, have a higher risk of all-cause mortality, compared with patients without tricuspid valvular disease [43]. Asymptomatic patients with HFpEF, but with severe aortic regurgitation (AR), have a higher risk of fatal cardiac events [44].

Comorbidities are very important in HF. Thus, comorbidity management plays a leading role in the treatment and progression of heart failure.

COPD is significantly more prevalent in HFrEF in our population. COPD and OSAS have common pathophysiological mechanisms, such as activation of sympathetic nervous system and inflammation, which can lead to increased cardiovascular risk. Furthermore, patients with association of these diseases, so called "overlap syndrome", are exposed to an even greater risk [7].

Some patients with advanced stages of COPD have right HF with peripheral edema and have increased likelihood of OSAS because of the shift of the rostral fluid from the legs during the night [45].

Chronic kidney disease is significantly more prevalent in the group of HFmrEF. Reports from ESADA (Sleep apnea network/European sleep apnea database) cohort study identify that in OSAS patients, decrease of GFR was predicted by baseline characteristics like older age, female gender, obese patients and severe nocturnal hypoxemia and by comorbidities like heart failure and arterial hypertension [46].

Several studies reported that HFmrEF patients have an increased risk of CAD as HFrEF patients, but all-cause mortality was similar to HFpEF [47,48]. The prognosis of HF, regardless of EF, was correlated with common risk factors, such as age, underlying disease and comorbidities [49].

Chioncel et al. found that the long-term mortality rate in HFmrEF was between those patients with HFpEF and HFrEF [50], whereas Pascual-Figa et al. showed that HFmrEF patients match a clinical profile similar to HFrEF, with an increased risk of cardiovascular mortality, rather than HFpEF [51]. Still, there are contradictory data from other recent studies which showed that HFmrEF patients have a prognosis similar to HFpEF patients [52,53]. The results of treatment in the latest publication show increased controversies [54].

5. Study Limitations

This study has several limitations. The studied population is relatively small, and even smaller for the subjects with HFrEF. There are no data about sleep since we did not perform full-night assisted polysomnography. The results need to be confirmed by larger studies.

6. Conclusions

Patients with OSAS and HF with mid-range EF may represent a new group of patients with increased risk of developing life-long chronic kidney disease, diabetes mellitus, and tricuspid and aortic insufficiency. COPD, myocardial infarction, impaired heart parietal kinetics and CAD are the most prevalent comorbidities in HFrEF patients, but the prevalence of these is closer to that of HFmrEF than HFpEF. More studies are needed, on larger groups of patients, to determine how OSAS is involved in the progression of HF, from borderline ejection fraction to more severe heart failure.

Author Contributions: Data curation, C.L.A., R.P., S.P., D.F.L., S.M.; formal analysis, S.U. and V.N.; methodology, C.L.A., S.P., D.F.L., S.M.; supervision, S.P., D.F.L., S.M.; writing—original draft, C.L.A., R.P., S.M.; writing—review and editing, C.L.A., S.P., S.M.

Funding: This research received no external funding.

Conflicts of Interest: The authors declare no conflict of interest.

References

1. Randerath, W.; Bassetti, C.L.; Bonsignore, M.R.; Farre, R.; Ferini-Strambi, L.; Grote, L.; Hedner, J.; Kohler, M.; Martinez-Garcia, M.A.; Mihaicuta, S.; et al. Challenges and perspectives in obstructive sleep apnea: Report by an ad hoc working group of the Sleep Disordered Breathing Group of the European Respiratory Society and the European Sleep Research Society. *Eur. Respir. J.* **2018**, *52*, 1702616. [CrossRef] [PubMed]
2. Yumino, D.; Wang, H.; Floras, J.S.; Newton, G.E.; Mak, S.; Ruttanaumpawan, P.; Parker, J.D.; Bradley, T.D. Prevalence and Physiological Predictors of Sleep Apnea in Patients With Heart Failure and Systolic Dysfunction. *J. Card. Fail.* **2009**, *15*, 279–285. [CrossRef] [PubMed]
3. Bassetti, C.L.; Milanova, M.; Gugger, M. Sleep-disordered breathing and acute ischemic stroke: Diagnosis, risk factors, treatment, evolution, and long-term clinical outcome. *Stroke* **2006**, *37*, 967–972. [CrossRef] [PubMed]
4. Logan, A.G.; Perlikowski, S.M.; Mente, A.; Tisler, A.; Tkacova, R.; Niroumand, M.; Leung, R.S.T.; Bradley, T.D. High prevalence of unrecognized sleep apnea in drug-resistant hypertension. *J. Hypertens.* **2001**, *19*, 2271–2277. [CrossRef] [PubMed]
5. Wang, H.; Parker, J.D.; Newton, G.E.; Floras, J.S.; Mak, S.; Chiu, K.-L.; Ruttanaumpawan, P.; Tomlinson, G.; Bradley, T.D. Influence of Obstructive Sleep Apnea on Mortality in Patients With Heart Failure. *J. Am. Coll. Cardiol.* **2007**, *49*, 1625–1631. [CrossRef] [PubMed]
6. Macdonald, M.; Fang, J.; Pittman, S.D.; White, D.P.; Malhotra, A. The Current Prevalence of Sleep Disordered Breathing in Congestive Heart Failure Patients Treated with Beta-Blockers. *J. Clin. Sleep Med.* **2008**, *4*, 38–42. [PubMed]
7. McNicholas, W.T.; Bonsignore, M.R. Sleep apnea as an independent risk factor for cardiovascular disease: Current evidence, basic mechanisms and research priorities. *Eur. Respir. J.* **2007**, *29*, 156–178. [CrossRef]
8. Bradley, T.D.; Floras, J.S. Sleep apnea and heart failure: Part I: Obstructive sleep apnea. *Circulation* **2003**, *107*, 1671–1678. [CrossRef]
9. Randerath, W.; Javaheri, S. Sleep-Disordered Breathing in Patients with Heart Failure. *Curr. Sleep Med. Rep.* **2016**, *2*, 99–106. [CrossRef]
10. Levy, P.; Kohler, M.; McNicholas, W.T.; Barbe, F.; McEvoy, R.D.; Somers, V.K.; Lavie, L.; Pepi, J.L. Obstructive sleep apnea syndrome. *Nat. Rev. Dis. Primers* **2015**, *1*, 15015. [CrossRef]
11. Mihaicuta, S.; Udrescu, M.; Topirceanu, A.; Udrescu, L. Network science meets respiratory medicine for OSAS phenotyping and severity prediction. *PeerJ* **2017**, *5*, e3289. [CrossRef]
12. Bonsignore, M.R.; Giron, M.C.S.; Marrone, O.; Castrogiovanni, A.; Montserrat, J.M. Personalised medicine in sleep respiratory disorders: Focus on obstructive sleep apnoea diagnosis and treatment. *Eur. Respir. Rev.* **2017**, *26*, 170069. [CrossRef]
13. Saaresranta, T.; Hedner, J.; Bonsignore, M.R.; Riha, R.L.; McNicholas, W.T.; Penzel, T.; Anttalainen, U.; Kvamme, J.A.; Pretl, M.; Sliwinski, P.; et al. Clinical Phenotypes and Comorbidity in European Sleep Apnoea Patients. *PLoS ONE* **2016**, *11*, e0163439. [CrossRef]
14. Van Riet, E.E.; Hoes, A.W.; Wagenaar, K.P.; Limburg, A.; Landman, M.A.; Rutten, F.H. Epidemiology of heart failure: The prevalence of heart failure and ventricular dysfunction in older adults over time. A systematic review. *Eur. J. Heart Fail.* **2016**, *18*, 242–252. [CrossRef]
15. Randerath, W.; Verbraecken, J.; Andreas, S.; Arzt, M.; Bloch, K.E.; Brack, T.; Buyse, B.; De Backer, W.; Eckert, D.J.; Grote, L.; et al. Definition, discrimination, diagnosis and treatment of central breathing disturbances during sleep. *Eur. Respir. J.* **2017**, *49*, 1600959. [CrossRef]

16. Butler, J.; Fonarow, G.C.; Zile, M.R.; Lam, C.S.; Roessig, L.; Schelbert, E.B.; Shah, S.J.; Ahmed, A.; Bonow, R.O.; Cleland, J.G.; et al. Developing Therapies for Heart Failure with Preserved Ejection Fraction: Current State and Future Directions. *JACC Hear. Fail.* **2014**, *2*, 97–112. [CrossRef]
17. Ponikowski, P.; Voors, A.A.; Anker, S.D.; Bueno, H.; Cleland, J.G.F.; Coats, A.J.S.; Falk, V.; González-Juanatey, J.R.; Harjola, V.P.; Jankowska, E.A.; et al. ESC Scientific Document Group; 2016 ESC Guidelines for the diagnosis and treatment of acute and chronic heart failure: The Task Force for the diagnosis and treatment of acute and chronic heart failure of the European Society of Cardiology (ESC) Developed with the special contribution of the Heart Failure Association (HFA) of the ESC. *Eur. Heart J.* **2016**, *37*, 2129–2200.
18. Fischer, J.; Dogas, Z.; Bassetti, C.L.; Berg, S.; Grote, L.; Jennum, P.; Levy, P.; Mihaicuta, S.; Nobili, L.; Riemann, D.; et al. Standard procedures for adults in accredited sleep medicine centres in Europe. Executive Committee of the Assembly of the National Sleep Societies; Board of the European Sleep Research Society, Regensburg, Germany. *J. Sleep Res.* **2012**, *21*, 357–368. [CrossRef]
19. Grigg-Damberger, M.M. The AASM Scoring Manual four years later. *J. Clin. Sleep Med.* **2012**, *8*, 597–619. [CrossRef]
20. Levey, A.S.; Stevens, L.A.; Schmid, C.H.; Zhang, Y.L.; Castro, A.F., 3rd; Feldman, H.I.; Kusek, J.W.; Eggers, P.; Van Lente, F.; Greene, T.; et al. A new equation to estimate glomerular filtration rate. *Ann. Intern Med.* **2009**, *150*, 604–612. [CrossRef]
21. Rudski, L.G.; Lai, W.W.; Afilalo, J.; Hua, L.; Handschumacher, M.D.; Chandrasekaran, K.; Solomon, S.D.; Louie, E.K.; Schiller, N.B. Guidelines for the echocardiographic assessment of the right heart in adults: A report from the American Society of Echocardiography endorsed by the European Association of Echocardiography, a registered branch of the European Society of Cardiology, and the Canadian Society of Echocardiography. *J. Am. Soc. Echocardiogr.* **2010**, *23*, 685–713, quiz: 786–788.
22. Lancellotti, P.; Tribouilloy, C.; Hagendorff, A.; Moura, L.; Popescu, B.A.; Agricola, E.; Monin, J.-L.; Pierard, L.A.; Badano, L.; Zamorano, J.L.; et al. European Association of Echocardiography recommendations for the assessment of valvular regurgitation. Part 1: Aortic and pulmonary regurgitation (native valve disease). *Eur. J. Echocardiogr.* **2010**, *11*, 223–244. [CrossRef]
23. Cheng, R.K.; Cox, M.; Neely, M.L.; Heidenreich, P.A.; Bhatt, D.L.; Eapen, Z.J.; Hernandez, A.F.; Butler, J.; Yancy, C.W.; Fonarow, G.C. Outcomes in patients with heart failure with preserved, borderline, and reduced ejection fraction in the Medicare population. *Am. Hear. J.* **2014**, *168*, 721–730. [CrossRef]
24. Kapoor, J.R.; Kapoor, R.; Ju, C.; Heidenreich, P.A.; Eapen, Z.J.; Hernandez, A.F.; Butler, J.; Yancy, C.W.; Yancy, G.C. Precipitating clinical factors, heart failure characterization, and outcomes in patients hospitalized with heart failure with reduced, borderline, and preserved ejection fraction. *JACC Heart Fail.* **2016**, *4*, 464–472. [CrossRef]
25. Tsuji, K.; Sakata, Y.; Nochioka, K.; Miura, M.; Yamauchi, T.; Onose, T.; Abe, R.; Oikawa, T.; Kasahara, S.; Sato, M.; et al. Characterization of heart failure patients with mid-range left ventricular ejection fraction-a report from the CHART-2 Study. *Eur. J. Hear. Fail.* **2017**, *19*, 1258–1269. [CrossRef]
26. Coles, A.H.; Tisminetzky, M.; Yarzebski, J.; Lessard, D.; Gore, J.M.; Darling, C.E.; Goldberg, R.J. Magnitude of and Prognostic Factors Associated With 1-Year Mortality after Hospital Discharge for Acute Decompensated Heart Failure Based on Ejection Fraction Findings. *J. Am. Heart Assoc.* **2015**, *4*, e002303. [CrossRef]
27. Gottlieb, D.J.; Yenokyan, G.; Newman, A.B.; O'Connor, G.T.; Punjabi, N.M.; Quan, S.F.; Redline, S.; Resnick, H.E.; Tong, E.K.; Diener-West, M.; et al. A Prospective Study of Obstructive Sleep Apnea and Incident Coronary Heart Disease and Heart Failure: The Sleep Heart Health Study. *Circulation* **2010**, *122*, 352–360. [CrossRef]
28. Perk, J.; De Backer, G.; Gohlke, H.; Graham, I.; Reiner, Z.; Verschuren, M.; Albus, C.; Benlian, P.; Boysen, G.; Cifkova, R.; et al. European Guidelines on cardiovascular disease prevention in clinical practice (version 2012). The Fifth Joint Task Force of the European Society of Cardiology and Other Societies on Cardiovascular Disease Prevention in Clinical Practice. *Eur. Heart J.* **2012**, *33*, 1635–1701.
29. Yumino, D.; Kasai, T.; Kimmerly, D.; Amirthalingam, V.; Floras, J.S.; Bradley, T.D. Differing Effects of Obstructive and Central Sleep Apneas on Stroke Volume in Patients with Heart Failure. *Am. J. Respir. Crit. Care Med.* **2013**, *187*, 433–438. [CrossRef]

30. Arzt, M.; Young, T.; Finn, L.; Skatrud, J.B.; Ryan, C.M.; Newton, G.E.; Mak, S.; Parker, J.D.; Floras, J.S.; Bradley, T.D. Sleepiness and sleep in patients with both systolic heart failure and obstructive sleep apnea. *Arch. Intern. Med.* **2006**, *166*, 1716–1722. [CrossRef]
31. Marin, J.M.; Carrizo, S.J.; Vicente, E.; Agusti, A.G. Long-term cardiovascular outcomes in men with obstructive sleep apnoea-hypopnoea with or without treatment with continuous positive airway pressure: An observational study. *Lancet* **2005**, *365*, 1046–1053. [CrossRef]
32. Reuter, H.; Herkenrath, S.; Treml, M.; Halbach, M.; Steven, D.; Frank, K.; Castrogiovanni, A.; Kietzmann, I.; Baldus, S.; Randerath, W.J. Sleep-disordered breathing in patients with cardiovascular diseases cannot be detected by ESS, STOP-BANG, and Berlin questionnaires. *Clin. Res. Cardiol.* **2018**, *107*, 1071–1078. [CrossRef]
33. Topîrceanu, A.; Udrescu, M.; Udrescu, L.; Ardelean, C.; Dan, R.; Reisz, D.; Mihaicuta, S. SAS score: Targeting high-specificity for efficient population-wide monitoring of obstructive sleep apnea. *PLoS ONE* **2018**, *13*, e0202042. [CrossRef]
34. Nielson, C.; Lange, T. Blood Glucose and Heart Failure in Nondiabetic Patients. *Diabetes Care* **2005**, *28*, 607–611. [CrossRef]
35. Udani, S.M.; Koyner, J.L. The Effects of Heart Failure on Renal Function. *Cardiol. Clin.* **2010**, *28*, 453–465. [CrossRef]
36. Marrone, O.; Bonsignore, M.R. Obstructive sleep apnea and chronic kidney disease: Open questions on a potential public health problem. *J. Thorac. Dis.* **2018**, *10*, 45–48. [CrossRef]
37. Agrawal, V.; Vanhecke, T.E.; Rai, B.; Franklin, B.A.; Sangal, R.B.; McCullough, P.A. Albuminuria and Renal Function in Obese Adults Evaluated for Obstructive Sleep Apnea. *Nephron Clin. Pr.* **2009**, *113*, c140–c147. [CrossRef]
38. Fleischmann, G.; Fillafer, G.; Matterer, H.; Skrabal, F.; Kotanko, P. Prevalence of chronic kidney disease in patients with suspected sleep apnea. *Nephrol. Dial. Transplant.* **2010**, *25*, 181–186. [CrossRef]
39. Gündüz, C.; Basoglu, O.K.; Hedner, J.; Zou, D.; Bonsignore, M.R.; Hein, H.; Staats, R.; Pataka, A.; Barbe, F.; Sliwinski, P.; et al. Obstructive sleep apnea independently predicts lipid levels: Data from the European Sleep Apnea Database. *Respirology* **2018**, *23*, 1180–1189. [CrossRef]
40. Holtstrand Hjälm, H.; Fu, M.; Hansson, P.O.; Zhong, Y.; Caidahl, K.; Mandalenakis, Z.; Morales, D.; Ergatoudes, C.; Rosengren, A.; Grote, L.; et al. Association between left atrial enlargement and obstructive sleep apnea in a general population of 71-year-old men. *J. Sleep Res.* **2018**, *27*, 252–258. [CrossRef]
41. Takemoto, Y.; Barnes, M.E.; Seward, J.B.; Lester, S.J.; Appleton, C.A.; Gersh, B.J.; Bailey, K.R.; Tsang, T.S. Usefulness of Left Atrial Volume in Predicting First Congestive Heart Failure in Patients ≥65 Years of Age With Well-Preserved Left Ventricular Systolic Function. *Am. J. Cardiol.* **2005**, *96*, 832–836. [CrossRef]
42. Hoit, B.D. Left Atrial Size and Function: Role in Prognosis. *J. Am. Coll. Cardiol.* **2014**, *63*, 493–505. [CrossRef]
43. Wang, N.; Fulcher, J.; Abeysuriya, N.; McGrady, M.; Wilcox, I.; Celermajer, D.; Lal, S. Tricuspid regurgitation is associated with increased mortality independent of pulmonary pressures and right heart failure: A systematic review and meta-analysis. *Eur. Heart J.* **2018**, *40*, 476–484. [CrossRef]
44. Detaint, D.; Messika-Zeitoun, D.; Maalouf, J.; Tribouilloy, C.; Mahoney, D.W.; Tajik, A.J.; Enriquez-Sarano, M. Quantitative echocardiographic determinants of clinical outcome in asymptomatic patients with aortic regurgitation: A prospective study. *JACC Cardiovasc. Imaging* **2008**, *1*, 1–11. [CrossRef]
45. McNicholas, W.T. Comorbid obstructive sleep apnea and chronic obstructive pulmonary disease and the risk of cardiovascular disease. *J. Thorac. Dis.* **2018**, *10*, S4253–S4261. [CrossRef]
46. Marrone, O.; Battaglia, S.; Steiropoulos, P.; Basoglu, O.K.; Kvamme, J.A.; Ryan, S.; Pepin, J.L.; Verbraecken, J.; Grote, L.; Hedner, J.; et al. ESADA study group. Chronic kidney disease in European patients with obstructive sleep apnea: The ESADA cohort study. *J. Sleep Res.* **2016**, *25*, 739–745. [CrossRef]
47. Vedin, O.; Lam, C.S.; Koh, A.S.; Benson, L.; Teng, T.H.K.; Tay, W.T.; Braun, O.Ö.; Savarese, G.; Dahlström, U.; Lund, L.H. Significance of ischemic heart disease in patients with heart failure and preserved, midrange, and reduced ejection fraction: A nationwide cohort study. *Circulation* **2017**, *10*, e003875. [CrossRef]
48. Wang, N.; Hales, S.; Barin, E.; Tofler, G. Characteristics and outcome for heart failure patients with mid-range ejection fraction. *J. Cardiovasc. Med.* **2018**, *19*, 297–303. [CrossRef]
49. Lam, C.S.; Gamble, G.D.; Ling, L.H.; Sim, D.; Leong, K.T.G.; Yeo, P.S.D.; Ong, H.Y.; Jaufeerally, F.; Ng, T.P.; Cameron, V.A.; et al. Mortality associated with heart failure with preserved vs. reduced ejection fraction in a prospective international multi-ethnic cohort study. *Eur. Heart J.* **2018**, *39*, 1770–1780. [CrossRef]

50. Chioncel, O.; Lainscak, M.; Seferovic, P.M.; Anker, S.D.; Crespo-Leiro, M.G.; Harjola, V.-P.; Parissis, J.; Laroche, C.; Piepoli, M.F.; Fonseca, C.; et al. Epidemiology and one-year outcomes in patients with chronic heart failure and preserved, mid-range and reduced ejection fraction: An analysis of the ESC Heart Failure Long-Term Registry. *Eur. J. Hear. Fail.* **2017**, *19*, 1574–1585. [CrossRef]
51. Pascual-Figal, D.A.; Ferrero-Gregori, A.; Gomez-Otero, I.; Vazquez, R.; Delgado-Jimenez, J.; Alvarez-Garcia, J.; Gimeno-Blanes, J.R.; Worner-Diz, F.; Bardají, A.; Alonso-Pulpon, L.; et al. MUSIC and REDINSCOR I research groups. Mid-range left ventricular ejection fraction: Clinical profile and cause of death in ambulatory patients with chronic heart failure. *Int. J. Cardiol.* **2017**, *240*, 265–270. [CrossRef] [PubMed]
52. Guisado-Espartero, M.E.; Salamanca-Bautista, P.; Aramburu-Bodas, Ó.; Conde-Martel, A.; Arias-Jiménez, J.L.; Llàcer-Iborra, P.; Dávila-Ramos, M.F.; Cabanes-Hernández, Y.; Manzano, L.; Montero-Pérez-Barquero, M.; et al. Heart failure with mid-range ejection fraction in patients admitted to internal medicine departments: Findings from the RICA registry. *Int. J. Cardiol.* **2018**, *255*, 124–128. [CrossRef] [PubMed]
53. Koh, A.S.; Tay, W.T.; Teng, T.H.K.; Vedin, O.; Benson, L.; Dahlström, U.; Savarese, G.; Lam, C.S.P.; Lund, L.H. A comprehensive population-based characterization of heart failure with mid-range ejection fraction. *Eur. J. Heart Fail.* **2017**, *19*, 1624–1634. [CrossRef] [PubMed]
54. McNicholas, W.T.; Bassetti, C.L.; Ferini-Strambi, L.; Pépin, J.L.; Pevernagie, D.; Verbraecken, J.; Randerath, W.; Baveno Working Group Members. Challenges in obstructive sleep apnoea. *Lancet Respir. Med.* **2018**, *6*, 170–172, Erratum in: *Lancet Respir. Med.* **2018**, *6*, e15. No abstract available. [CrossRef]

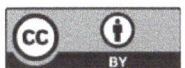

© 2019 by the authors. Licensee MDPI, Basel, Switzerland. This article is an open access article distributed under the terms and conditions of the Creative Commons Attribution (CC BY) license (http://creativecommons.org/licenses/by/4.0/).

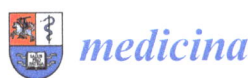

Article

Magnitude and Determinants of Patients at Risk of Developing Obstructive Sleep Apnea in a Non-Communicable Disease Clinic

Prakash Mathiyalagen [1], Venkatesh Govindasamy [2,*], Anandaraj Rajagopal [1], Kavita Vasudevan [1], Kalaipriya Gunasekaran [1] and Dhananjay Yadav [3,*]

1. Department of Community Medicine, Indira Gandhi Medical College & Research Institute, Kathirkamam, Vazhudavur Road, Puducherry 605010, India
2. Department of Community Medicine, Government Thiruvannamalai Medical College & Hospital, Thiruvannamalai 606604, India
3. Department of Medical Biotechnology, Yeungnam University, Gyeongsan 38541, Korea
* Correspondence: drvenkat90021@gmail.com (V.G.); dhanyadav16481@gmail.com (D.Y.); Tel.: +91-9894597687 (V.G.); +82-1022021191 (D.Y.)

Received: 12 May 2019; Accepted: 16 July 2019; Published: 20 July 2019

Abstract: *Background and Objective*: Obstructive sleep apnea (OSA) is a common chronic disorder worldwide, which can adversely affect the cardiovascular system among non-communicable disease (NCD) patients. It is underdiagnosed—or rather not diagnosed—in primary care settings due to the costly diagnostic techniques involved. This study aimed to assess the number of study participants at risk of developing OSA and to assess and quantify the risk factors associated with this disorder. *Materials and Methods*: A cross-sectional study was performed in an NCD clinic of a rural health training center, Karikalampakkam, Puducherry of South India from August 2018 to October 2018. A Modified Berlin Questionnaire (MBQ) was used to screen the study participants at risk for OSA. Four-hundred-and-seventy-three people aged 18 years and above were included in the study, using systematic random sampling. Respondents' socio-demographic and morbidity characteristics, as well as clinical and anthropometric parameters including body weight, height, blood pressure, neck, hip and waist circumference were collected. Data was captured using Epicollect5 and analyzed using SPSS version 20.0. *Results*: One-fourth (25.8%) of the respondents were at high risk of developing OSA. In terms of gender, 27.9% of the men and 23.8% of the women were at high risk for OSA. In univariate analyses, the risk of developing OSA was significantly associated with a history of diabetes mellitus, hypertension, dyslipidemia and gastro-esophageal reflux disease, weight, body mass index, neck, waist and hip circumference, waist–hip ratio, and systolic and diastolic blood pressure. Multivariate logistic regression analysis showed that a history of dyslipidemia (aOR, 95% CI = 2.34, 1.22–4.48), body mass index (aOR, 95% CI = 1.15, 1.06–1.22) and waist circumference (aOR, 95% CI = 1.10, 1.07–1.14) emerged as significant predictors of risk for OSA. *Conclusions*: A considerable proportion of NCD patients with easily detectable attributes are at risk of developing OSA, but still remain undiagnosed at a primary health care setting. The results obtained using MBQ in this study were comparable to studies performed using polysomnography. Dyslipidemia, body mass index and waist circumference were independent risk factors for predicting a risk of developing OSA. Prospective studies are needed to confirm whether a reduction in these risk factors could reduce the risk for OSA.

Keywords: obstructive sleep apnea; non-communicable disease; Modified Berlin Questionnaire; dyslipidemia; body mass index; waist circumference

1. Introduction

Obstructive sleep apnoea (OSA) is a common disorder, characterized by repeated episodes of a complete or partial collapse of the upper airway (chiefly the oropharyngeal tract) at the time of sleep, with a subsequent reduction of the airflow [1]. In India, OSA prevalence varies from 9.3% to 13.7% [2,3]. The causes of developing OSA are multifactorial, comprising of a multifaceted interaction between anatomic, neuromuscular issues, along with an underlying genetic predisposition toward the disease [4]. The risk factors consist of snoring, a male gender, middle age, menopausal women, obesity and a range of craniofacial and oropharyngeal structures such as a bulky neck circumference, retro-or micrognazia, a nasal impediment, expended tonsils, and a low-lying soft palate [4,5].

As the ailment advancements, the sleepiness gradually becomes dangerous, resulting in reduced accomplishments at work and major job- and road-related mishaps [6]. Furthermore, many patients can suffer from cognitive and neurobehavioral impairment, an inability to concentrate, memory loss and mood variations such as irritability and depression. This further disrupts a person's performance at work with significant results [7]. Sleep-related hypoxia has been linked with a systemic inflammation that may contribute to the commencement or quickening of the process of atherogenesis [8]. In addition, a significant metabolic deterioration arises in OSA independently from weight [6]. Insulin resistance, type 2 diabetes, and disturbed serum lipid parameters—broadly observed in patients with OSA—further increase in risk of cardiovascular illness [6,9–11].

Regrettably, numerous sufferers of OSA are undiagnosed [12]. This is likely because the standard measurement for diagnosis is overnight polysomnography (PSG) which is costly and not generally available [13]. Likewise, the attendant uneasiness of patients spending the whole night in sleep laboratories makes it rather impractical for large numbers of patients—whether as a diagnostic measurement tool or as a screening protocol [13].

A reasonable explanation for the foregoing difficulties in sleep study has been the advancement of questionnaires estimating sleep-related disorders and OSA [14]. Previous studies have utilized the standardized questionnaires like the Epworth sleepiness scale (ESS), the STOP (snoring, tiredness, observed apnea, high blood pressure) questionnaire, and the Cleveland sleep habits questionnaire (CSHQ) [13–15]. Still, the Berlin Questionnaire (BQ) remains the most extensively used screening questionnaire for OSA [15]. A Modified Berlin Questionnaire has been developed to suit Asian populations. Previously, the predictive value of the Modified Berlin Questionnaire for identifying the risk of developing OSA has been analyzed by using the receiver operating characteristic (ROC) curve, that resulted in a sensitivity of 85% and specificity of 95%. The positive predictive value was 96% and the negative predictive value was 82%. Questions about the symptoms demonstrated internal consistency (Cronbach α correlations 0.92–0.96) [16].

Research conducted in developed countries to illustrate and establish the risk factors linked with OSA reported that few of the risk factors are preventable [6,17,18]. Therefore, in this study, we focused on assessing and quantifying the risk factors associated with OSA and estimating the proportion of study participants who are at high risk of developing OSA, visiting an NCD clinic in a rural health training center attached to a tertiary care hospital of Puducherry, using the Modified Berlin Questionnaire. Additionally, we analyzed the cut-off value of waist circumference and BMI to predict the risk of developing OSA in the recruited subjects.

2. Materials and Methods

2.1. Study Setting

This facility-based cross-sectional study was undertaken in a peripheral health care setting from August 2018 to October 2018, among patients attending a non-communicable disease clinic. The rural health training centre (RHTC), Karikalampakkam, is one of the field practice areas of the department of community medicine—Indira Gandhi Medical College and Research Institute—located in the Union Territory of Puducherry, India. This RHTC caters for a population of around 37,000.

Non-communicable disease clinics are conducted on a bi-weekly basis where new (i.e., referred from an out-patient department and an in-patient department) and old diabetic, hypertensive and cardiac cases come for a regular check-up as well as to collect their medication. Routinely, between 150 and 200 NCD patients are seen in a single NCD clinic day.

2.2. Inclusion Criteria

All Patients more than or equal to 18 years of age and less than or equal to 70 years attending NCD clinic for the first time during the study period were included in the study.

2.3. Exclusion Criteria

Those with inadequate time (<6 h) in bed for sleeping (as adequate sleep is defined as between 6 and 8 h per night regularly) [19–23], extraneous sleep disruption (e.g., babies/children) and with shift work were excluded from the study.

2.4. Sample Size Estimation

Considering that the prevalence of OSA among the adult population is 13.7% [3], and taking the alpha error as 5% and absolute error of margin as 5%, the minimum sample size was calculated as 185. With the design effect of 2 for this systematic random sampling technique and the 10% non-response rate, we decided to take a minimum of 410 samples.

2.5. Sampling Technique

The study was conducted by interviewing every 3rd patient attending the NCD clinic following systematic random sampling.

2.6. Study Tool

The study participants were interviewed using a pre-tested semi-structured questionnaire, with questions on socio-demographic data, anthropometric data for assessing risk factors and the Modified Berlin questionnaire [16] for screening OSA. Physical parameters like height, weight, neck circumference, waist circumference, hip circumference, and BP were measured using standard procedures. A score of 2 or more positive categories indicates a high risk for OSA syndrome and only 1 or no positive category indicates a low risk for OSA syndrome.

2.7. Ethics

The data collection began after obtaining permission from the Institutional Ethics Committee located in Indira Gandhi Medical College & Research Institute, Kathirkamam, Puducherry, with its approval letter No. 17/IEC/IGMC/F-7/2017/28 dated 12 August 2017. Informed written consent was obtained from the study participants after explaining the objectives of the study.

2.8. Statistical Methods

The data was collected using epicollect5 and analyzed using Epi-info and SPSS version 20. The normality of the data distribution was assessed using the Shapiro–Wilk Test. Since the p value of the Shapiro–Wilk Test was greater than 0.05, the data distribution was normal and parametric tests were applied. The quantitative data was represented as mean and standard deviation and the qualitative data was described by proportions and percentages. The chi-squared test and Student t-test were used based on the data variables. A binomial logistic regression analysis was performed to determine the confounding factors and find the adjusted odds' ratio. A receiver operating a characteristic curve analysis with the Youden index J statistic was performed to assess the optimal cut-off point for the significant anthropometric indices predicting risks of developing OSA. A p value of less than 0.05 was considered statistically significant.

3. Results

A total of 473 NCD patients participated in this study. The mean age of the study participants was 51 ± 11.34 years. The descriptive profile and univariate analyses of the study subjects are shown in Table 1. About 51% of the study subjects were males and so the male–female proportion is almost equal. The majority (67%) were less than 60 years old. Most of them (85%) were married. Almost 54% were sedentary workers, while the remainder were either moderate workers or heavy workers. A majority (75%) were non-smokers and non-drinkers of alcohol. About half of them were diabetic and hypertensive, and more than 15% had higher blood cholesterol and respiratory illness. Table 1 gives the association of socio-demographic and morbidity factors with risks of developing OSA. Among the study participants, 25.8% had a high risk of developing OSA based on the modified Berlin questionnaire criteria. From this study, it was found that a history of diabetes mellitus, hypertension, dyslipidemia and GERD were significantly associated with a greater risk of developing OSA.

Table 1. Association of socio-demographic and morbidity factors with risks of developing obstructive sleep apnea (OSA) (n = 473).

Variable	High Risk for OSA (%)	Low Risk for OSA (%)	p Value [#]	Unadjusted OR (95% CI)
Gender				
Male	64 (27.9)	165 (72.1)	0.299	1.244 (0.823–1.879)
Female	58 (23.8)	186 (76.2)		
Age				
</=60 years	84 (26.3)	235 (73.7)	0.700	1.091 (0.701–1.699)
>60 years	38 (24.7)	116 (75.3)		
Marital status				
Others (unmarried/widow/divorce)	20 (29.9)	47 (70.1)		
Married	102 (25.1)	304 (74.9)	0.413	1.268 (0.718–2.241)
Occupation				
Sedentary worker	66 (25.6)	192 (74.4)		
Moderate worker	47 (26.4)	131 (73.6)	0.847	0.958 (0.620–1.480) Ref
Heavy worker	9 (24.3)	28 (75.7)	0.870	1.069 (0.480–2.383) Ref
Smoking history				
Smoker	38 (31.9)	81 (68.1)	0.077	1.508 (0.955–2.381)
Non-smoker	84 (23.7)	270 (76.3)		
Alcohol history				
Drinker	36 (31.0)	80 (69.0)	0.137	1.418 (0.893–2.251)
Non-drinker	86 (24.1)	271 (75.9)		
History of diabetes mellitus				
Yes	75 (32.3)	157 (67.7)	0.001	1.972 (1.294–3.004)
No	47 (19.5)	194 (80.5)		
History of hypertension				
Yes	83 (31.0)	185 (69.0)	0.003	1.910 (1.237–2.948)
No	39 (19.0)	166 (81.0)		
History of Dyslipidemia				
Yes	32 (45.1)	39 (54.9)	<0.001	2.844 (1.686–4.799)
No	90 (22.4)	312 (77.6)		
History of Respiratory illness [*]				
Yes	24 (30.8)	54 (69.2)	0.272	1.347 (0.791–2.294)
No	98 (24.8)	297 (75.2)		
History of GERD				
Yes	32 (38.1)	52 (61.9)	0.004	2.044 (1.241–3.369)
No	90 (23.1)	299 (76.9)		
History of Sore throat				
Yes	10 (30.3)	23 (69.7)	0.539	1.273 (0.588–2.758)
No	112 (25.5)	328 (74.5)		

[*] Asthma/COPD; [#] Chi-square test; OR: odds ratio; CI: confidence interval; OSA: obstructive sleep apnoea; GERD: gastro-esophageal reflux disease.

The mean neck circumference, waist circumference and hip circumference of the study participants with a high risk of developing OSA was 37.26 ± 3.51 cm, 95.03 ± 8.49 cm and 104.47 ± 7.78 cm respectively. The mean waist–hip ratio among those with a high risk of developing OSA was 0.91, compared to a ratio of 0.89 among those with a low risk of developing OSA. The mean weight among those with a high risk of developing OSA (72.83 ± 10.75 kg) was a little higher than those with a low risk of developing OSA (63.83 ± 10.59 kg). As shown in Table 2, there was a statistically significant difference in the mean neck circumference, weight, body mass index, waist circumference, hip circumference, waist–hip ratio, systolic blood pressure and diastolic blood pressure between groups considered to be at a high risk and those considered to be at a low risk of developing OSA. In the univariate analyses, it was found that six out of seven anthropometric factors were significantly associated with a high risk of developing OSA.

Table 2. Association of clinical and anthropometric factors with risk for OSA (n = 473).

Variable	High Risk for OSA (N = 122) (Mean ± SD)	Low Risk for OSA (N = 351) (Mean ± SD)	p-Value $^\$$	Mean Difference (95% CI)
Neck circumference (cm)	37.26 (3.51)	36.18 (3.34)	0.003	1.080 (0.362–1.798)
Weight (kg)	72.83 (10.75)	63.83 (10.59)	<0.001	8.99 (6.77–11.21)
Height (cm)	159.20 (8.27)	158.08 (8.29)	0.198	1.12 (−0.59–2.84)
BMI (kg/sq.m)	28.81 (4.23)	25.57 (4.03)	<0.001	3.24 (2.37–4.11)
Waist circumference (cm)	95.03 (8.49)	86.62 (8.87)	<0.001	8.41 (6.63–10.19)
Hip circumference (cm)	104.47 (7.78)	97.40 (7.79)	<0.001	7.06 (5.45–8.67)
Systolic blood pressure (mmHg)	141.57 (14.86)	133.77 (15.75)	<0.001	7.81 (4.68–10.93)
Diastolic blood pressure (mmHg)	86.42 (9.00)	83.07 (10.49)	0.001	3.35 (1.40–5.30)
Waist Hip Ratio	0.911 (0.067)	0.892 (0.088)	0.015	0.019 (0.0037–0.0338)

$^\$$ Students t test; SD: standard deviation; CI: confidence interval; OSA: obstructive sleep apnoea; BMI: body mass index.

In Table 3, the variables which were found to be significant from the univariate analyses (p < 0.05) in Tables 1 and 2 were considered for binomial logistic regression analysis. However, on further analysis using binary logistic regression, only three risk factors were found to be associated significantly with a high risk of developing OSA. These were dyslipidemia (aOR 2.342, 95% CI 1.224–4.482), body mass index (aOR 1.147, 95% CI 1.075–1.223) and waist circumference (aOR 1.102, 95% CI 1.065–1.141), as presented in Table 3.

Table 3. Predictors of risk for OSA by binary logistic regression analysis (n = 473).

	B	S.E.	Wald	p-Value	Adjusted Odds Ratio (95% CI)
History of DM (No as reference)	0.380	0.252	2.274	0.132	1.462 (0.892–2.394)
History of Dyslipidemia (No as reference)	0.851	0.331	6.601	0.010	2.342 (1.224–4.482)
History of GERD (No as reference)	0.093	0.309	0.092	0.762	1.098 (0.600–2.010)
Neck circumference	0.017	0.037	0.210	0.647	1.017 (0.947–1.092)
Body mass index	0.137	0.033	17.344	0.000	1.147 (1.075–1.223)
Waist circumference	0.097	0.017	31.090	0.000	1.102 (1.065–1.141)
Systolic blood pressure	0.019	0.010	3.748	0.053	1.019 (1.000–1.038)
Diastolic blood pressure	−0.006	0.014	0.166	0.683	0.994 (0.968–1.021)
Constant	−16.670	2.248	54.985	0.000	0.000

OSA: obstructive sleep apnoea; B: estimated logit coefficient; SE: standard error of the coefficient; Wald: test statistic using chi-square test; CI: confidence interval; DM: diabetes mellitus; GERD: gastro-esophageal reflux disease.

As depicted in Table 4, the area under the ROC curve was statistically significant in terms of waist circumference and body mass index, and the cut-off value had a high level of predictive accuracy for detecting the risk of developing OSA in both genders. In Figure 1, the values 94.0 cm for waist circumference (sensitivity, 73%; specificity, 74%), and 24.0 kg/m² for body mass index (sensitivity, 94%; specificity, 44%) represented the optimum cut-off for males. In Figure 2, the values of 92 cm for waist circumference (sensitivity, 62%; specificity, 77%), and 27 kg/m² for body mass index (sensitivity, 78%; specificity, 60%) represented the optimum cut-off for females.

Table 4. Cut-off values for waist circumference and body mass index to predict the risk of developing OSA in males and females.

	Waist Circumference		Body Mass Index	
	Male	Female	Male	Female
Area under the ROC curve (95% CI)	0.79 (0.70–0.87)	0.74 (0.65–0.83)	0.74 (0.64–0.82)	0.73 (0.63–0.82)
p-value	<0.001	<0.001	<0.001	<0.001
Cut-off value	94.0 cm	92.0 cm	24.0 kg/m²	27.0 kg/m²
Sensitivity	73%	62%	94%	78%
Specificity	74%	77%	44%	60%

ROC curve: receiver operating characteristic curve; CI: confidence interval.

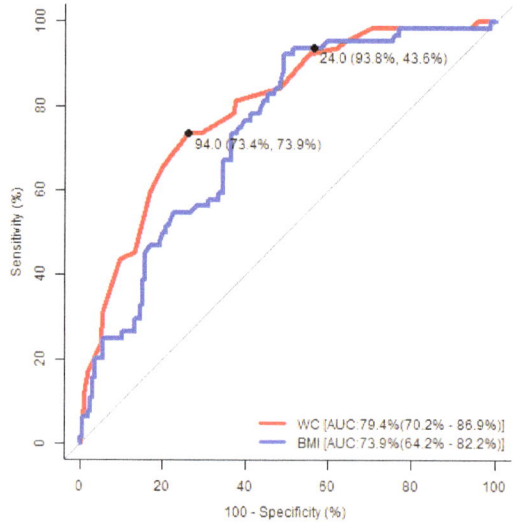

Figure 1. Receiver operating characteristic analysis to determine the optimal cut-off values of the significant anthropometric indices to predict the risk of developing obstructive sleep apnea (OSA) in males. WC: waist circumference; BMI: body mass index; AUC: area under the curve.

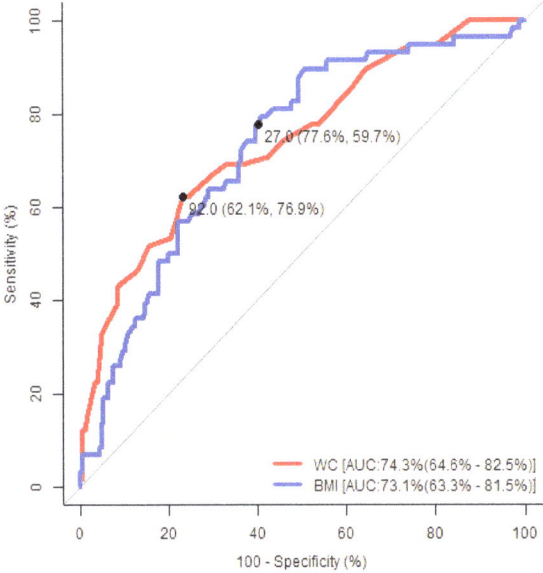

Figure 2. Receiver operating characteristic analysis to determine the optimal cut-off values of the significant anthropometric indices to predict the risk of developing obstructive sleep apnea (OSA) in females. WC: waist circumference; BMI: body mass index; AUC: area under the curve.

4. Discussion

This facility-based study was conducted among NCD clinic attendees in a rural health training center under a medical college in Puducherry, using a Modified Berlin questionnaire which is a widely used, validated, reliable and simple tool for predicting the risk of developing OSA [11,12]. The proportion of patients attending the NCD clinic who were at a high risk of developing OSA was found to be 25.8% in this study. Viswanathan et al. documented that 23.65% of the study subjects attending diabetic clinic in Chennai had OSA [24]. Though this study utilized the Apnea–Hypopnea Index (AHI) to determine OSA, the present questionnaire-based study result matches with the above findings. Rashid et al. reported that 19.4% of the primary care clinic attendees in Malaysia were at a high risk of developing OSA when assessed using the BQ [25]. The lower prevalence in that study could be due to the fact that all of the patients attending the hospital were randomly assessed, whereas the present study focused only on the NCD clinic attendees. The present study observed that males (27.9%) were at a higher risk of developing OSA compared to females (23.8%). Similarly, a higher male preponderance for developing OSA has been documented by different researchers [24,26].

Despite the biologic plausibility of an association between smoking and the development of OSA, and the high prevalence of both the disorders, there is no adequate evidence to establish a significant relationship clinically [27]. This finding from the systematic review agrees with our study results. Simou et al. stated in their meta-analysis that people who consumed alcohol were about 25% more likely to suffer from OSA [28]. Consumption of alcohol increases the risk of developing OSA by reducing genioglossal muscle tone, leading to upper airway collapse and increased upper airway resistance [28]. The present study exhibited an association, though not one which was statistically significant. The reason could be that their treatment for the non-communicable disease may have prevented them from consuming alcohol and smoking.

Huang et al. identified a bidirectional association between OSA and diabetes mellitus in a large population-based study [29]. A similar association has been observed in the present study in the univariate analyses. Recurrent catecholamine production due to recurrent hypoxemia in

OSA can impair glucose tolerance, reduce insulin sensitivity and cause type 2 diabetes mellitus [29]. Regarding diabetes mellitus and incident OSA, plausible factors like insulin resistance, leptin resistance, elevated systemic inflammatory metabolites and oxidative stress could reduce the airway response to hypercapnia, impair the neuromechanical control of airways and weaken the upper airway respiratory muscles—predisposing a person to developing OSA [29].

In a systematic review, Hou et al. reported that OSA and hypertension had a significant association [30], which corroborates the present study's findings in the univariate analyses. Intermittent hypoxia in recurrent OSA can upregulate the sympathetic nervous system and cause sustained hypertension [30,31].

Kim et al. ascertained that esophagogastroduodenoscopy-proven GERD was significantly associated with OSA, which substantiates our study's results. A recurrent upper airway narrowing among OSA patients during sleep could result in negative intra-thoracic pressure during inspiration [32]. The increased intrathoracic pressure might facilitate acid reflux into the esophagus, which finally leads to GERD [32]. GERD could deteriorate OSA by aggravating the airway resistance by causing posterior laryngitis [32].

The present study observed a strong association between dyslipidemia and OSA, which corroborates the findings which have been stated by Adedayo et al. in their systematic review [33]. Gündüz et al. observed a significant association between higher total cholesterol, higher LDL-cholesterol, elevated triglycerides, lower HDL-cholesterol and OSA [34]. Recurrent hypoxia during sleep in OSA patients could generate stearoyl-coenzyme A desaturase-1 and oxygen free radicals, leading to lipid peroxidation and eventually, dyslipidemia [33].

Kang HH et al. conducted a study among patients attending sleep clinics in Korea and found that the adjusted odds' ratio and 95% CI for body mass index, neck circumference and waist circumference were 1.364 (1.22–1.53), 1.414 (1.24–1.62) and 1.114 (1.07–1.16) respectively [35]. The present study identified a similar risk in the anthropometric indices, except for neck circumference, as this study was conducted in non-communicable disease clinic. In a study which was conducted among the Turkish population, Soylu et al. found that BMI values over 28.93 kg/m^2 in males and over 27.77 kg/m^2 in females increased the risk of developing OSA [36]. Kang HH et al. found, in a study which was conducted among the Korean population, that BMI values over 24.95 kg/m^2 in males and over 23.05 kg/m^2 in females increased the risk of developing OSA [35]. The cut-off value for BMI being a risk factor for the development of OSA was over 24.00 kg/m^2 in males and over 27.00 kg/m^2 in females in the present study. The waist circumference cut-off for predicting the risks of developing OSA mentioned by Kang HH et al. was >105 cm for males and >101 cm female [35], whereas the present study delivered figures of >94 cm for males and >92 cm for females. The reason for these variations in the cut-off points could be the regional and hormonal influence in determining these factors. Subramanian S et al. established a gender difference concerning the risk factors for developing OSA where females had a higher BMI, higher hip circumference, lower waist–hip ratio, thin neck circumference and similar waist circumference compared to males. The present study also found a gender difference which was documented in Figures 1 and 2, where a high BMI and similar waist circumference were observed among females compared to males as the cut-off to identify the risk of developing OSA [37].

This study has some limitations which must be discussed. First, because the current study was a cross-sectional study, the temporal association could not be assessed. Second, the predictive performance of modified BQ for the risk categorization of developing OSA, was not comparable to gold standard overnight polysomnography. This BQ has the highest sensitivity and specificity among the available tools for assessing the risk for OSA and is also a valid and reliable screening tool to be used in resource constraint settings. Third, the study subjects were taken from the NCD clinic and so generalizations had to be discussed based on these settings. Since non-communicable diseases have been escalating in India [38], the present study could show the magnitude and determinant factors of this neglected NCD.

5. Conclusions

OSA was determined as a common disorder among non-communicable disease patients, as it was observed in 27.9% and 23.8% of males and females, respectively. Dyslipidemia, body mass index and waist circumference were independent risk factors for predicting the risk of developing OSA, based on multivariate regression analysis. In addition, the present study reported the cut-off values of body mass index and waist circumference that increase the risk for OSA.

Author Contributions: Conceptualization, methodology, data curation P.M., V.G., A.R., K.V.; supervision P.M., K.G.; writing P.M., D.Y.; statistical analysis P.M., V.G., A.R., K.G., D.Y.

Funding: This research received no external funding.

Acknowledgments: The authors would like to thank all the study participants, interns, post-graduates and statistician for their contribution to this research.

Conflicts of Interest: The authors declare no conflict of interest.

References

1. Spicuzza, L.; Caruso, D.; Di Maria, G. Obstructive sleep apnoea syndrome and its management. *Ther. Adv. Chronic Dis.* **2015**, *6*, 273–285. [CrossRef] [PubMed]
2. Reddy, E.V.; Kadhiravan, T.; Mishra, H.K.; Sreenivas, V.; Handa, K.K.; Sinha, S.; Sharma, S.K. Prevalence and risk factors of obstructive sleep apnea among middle-aged urban Indians: A community-based study. *Sleep Med.* **2009**, *10*, 913–918. [CrossRef] [PubMed]
3. Sharma, S.K.; Kumpawat, S.; Banga, A.; Goel, A. Prevalence and risk factors of obstructive sleep apnea syndrome in a population of Delhi, India. *Chest* **2006**, *130*, 149–156. [CrossRef] [PubMed]
4. Dempsey, J.; Veasey, S.; Morgan, B.; O'Donnell, C. Pathophysiology of sleep apnea. *Physiol. Rev.* **2010**, *90*, 47–112. [CrossRef]
5. Ahmad, A.N.; McLeod, G.; Al Zahrani, N.; Al Zahrani, H. Screening for high risk of sleep apnea in an ambulatory care setting in saudi arabia. *Int. J. Environ. Res. Public Health* **2019**, *16*, 459. [CrossRef] [PubMed]
6. Jordan, A.S.; McSharry, D.G.; Malhotra, A. Adult obstructive sleep apnoea. *Lancet* **2014**, *383*, 736–747. [CrossRef]
7. Vaessen, T.J.; Overeem, S.; Sitskoorn, M.M. Cognitive complaints in obstructive sleep apnea. *Sleep Med. Rev.* **2015**, *19*, 51–58. [CrossRef]
8. Unnikrishnan, D.; Jun, J.; Polotsky, V. Inflammation in sleep apnea: An update. *Rev. Endocr. Metab. Disord.* **2015**, *16*, 25–34. [CrossRef]
9. Tahrani, A.A.; Ali, A. Obstructive sleep apnoea and type 2 diabetes. *Eur. Endocrinol.* **2014**, *10*, 43–50. [CrossRef]
10. Kent, B.D.; McNicholas, W.T.; Ryan, S. Insulin resistance, glucose intolerance and diabetes mellitus in obstructive sleep apnoea. *J. Thorac. Dis.* **2015**, *7*, 1343–1357.
11. Yadav, D.; Cho, K.H. Total sleep duration and risk of type 2 diabetes: Evidence-based on clinical and epidemiological studies. *Curr. Drug Metab.* **2018**, *19*, 979–985. [CrossRef] [PubMed]
12. Ulualp, S.O. Snoring and obstructive sleep apnea. *Med. Clin. N. Am.* **2010**, *94*, 1047–1055. [CrossRef] [PubMed]
13. Abrishami, A.; Khajehdehi, A.; Chung, F. A systematic review of screening questionnaires for obstructive sleep apnea. *Can. J. Anaesth. J. Can. d–Anesthesie* **2010**, *57*, 423–438. [CrossRef] [PubMed]
14. Senthilvel, E.; Auckley, D.; Dasarathy, J. Evaluation of sleep disorders in the primary care setting: History taking compared to questionnaires. *J. Clin. Sleep Med.* **2011**, *7*, 41–48. [PubMed]
15. Sogebi, O.A.; Ogunwale, A. Risk factors of obstructive sleep apnea among Nigerian outpatients. *Braz. J. Otorhinolaryngol.* **2012**, *78*, 27–33. [CrossRef] [PubMed]
16. Sharma, S.K.; Vasudev, C.; Sinha, S.; Banga, A.; Pandey, R.M.; Handa, K.K. Validation of the modified berlin questionnaire to identify patients at risk for the obstructive sleep apnoea syndrome. *Indian J. Med. Res.* **2006**, *124*, 281–290. [PubMed]
17. Yacoub, M.; Youssef, I.; Salifu, M.O.; McFarlane, S.I. Cardiovascular disease risk in obstructive sleep apnea: An update. *J. Sleep Disord. Ther.* **2017**, *7*, 283. [CrossRef] [PubMed]
18. Ahmad, M.; Makati, D.; Akbar, S. Review of and updates on hypertension in obstructive sleep apnea. *Int. J. Hypertens.* **2017**, *2017*, 1848375. [CrossRef]

19. Chen, M.-Y.; Wang, E.K.; Jeng, Y.-J. Adequate sleep among adolescents is positively associated with health status and health-related behaviors. *BMC Public Health* **2006**, *6*, 59. [CrossRef]
20. World Health Organization. Regional Office for Europe and the European Centre for Environment and Health Bonn Office. In Proceedings of the WHO Technical Meeting on Sleep and Health, Bonn, Germany, 22–24 January 2004.
21. Hirshkowitz, M.; Whiton, K.; Albert, S.M.; Alessi, C.; Bruni, O.; DonCarlos, L.; Hazen, N.; Herman, J.; Hillard, P.J.A.; Katz, E.S. National sleep foundation's updated sleep duration recommendations. *Sleep Health* **2015**, *1*, 233–243. [CrossRef]
22. Yadav, D.; Hyun, D.S.; Ahn, S.V.; Koh, S.B.; Kim, J.Y. A prospective study of the association between total sleep duration and incident hypertension. *J. Clin. Hypertens.* **2017**, *19*, 550–557. [CrossRef] [PubMed]
23. Kim, J.Y.; Yadav, D.; Ahn, S.V.; Koh, S.B.; Park, J.T.; Yoon, J.; Yoo, B.S.; Lee, S.H. A prospective study of total sleep duration and incident metabolic syndrome: The arirang study. *Sleep Med.* **2015**, *16*, 1511–1515. [CrossRef] [PubMed]
24. Viswanathan, V.; Ramalingam, I.P.; Ramakrishnan, N. High prevalence of obstructive sleep apnea among people with type 2 diabetes mellitus in a tertiary care center. *J. Assoc. Physicians India* **2017**, *65*, 38–42. [PubMed]
25. Rashid, R.; Ahmad, S.; Jaffar, A.; Ali, F.; Paidi, N. Determinants of patients at risk of developing obstructive sleep apnea in a primary care clinic. *Res. Updates Med. Sci.* **2014**, *2*, 70–74.
26. Kang, K.; Seo, J.-G.; Seo, S.-H.; Park, K.-S.; Lee, H.-W. Prevalence and related factors for high-risk of obstructive sleep apnea in a large Korean population: Results of a questionnaire-based study. *J. Clin. Neurol.* **2014**, *10*, 42–49. [CrossRef] [PubMed]
27. Krishnan, V.; Dixon-Williams, S.; Thornton, J.D. Where there is smoke ... there is sleep apnea: Exploring the relationship between smoking and sleep apnea. *Chest* **2014**, *146*, 1673–1680. [CrossRef] [PubMed]
28. Simou, E.; Britton, J.; Leonardi-Bee, J. Alcohol and the risk of sleep apnoea: A systematic review and meta-analysis. *Sleep Med.* **2018**, *42*, 38–46. [CrossRef] [PubMed]
29. Huang, T.; Lin, B.M.; Stampfer, M.J.; Tworoger, S.S.; Hu, F.B.; Redline, S. A population-based study of the bidirectional association between obstructive sleep apnea and type 2 diabetes in three prospective us cohorts. *Diabetes Care* **2018**, *41*, 2111–2119. [CrossRef]
30. Hou, H.; Zhao, Y.; Yu, W.; Dong, H.; Xue, X.; Ding, J.; Xing, W.; Wang, W. Association of obstructive sleep apnea with hypertension: A systematic review and meta-analysis. *J. Glob. Health* **2018**, *8*, 010405. [CrossRef]
31. McEvoy, R.D. Obstructive sleep apnoea and hypertension: The esada study. *Eur. Respir. J.* **2014**, *44*, 835–838. [CrossRef]
32. Kim, Y.; Lee, Y.J.; Park, J.S.; Cho, Y.-J.; Yoon, H.I.; Lee, J.H.; Lee, C.-T.; Kim, S.J. Associations between obstructive sleep apnea severity and endoscopically proven gastroesophageal reflux disease. *Sleep Breath.* **2018**, *22*, 85–90. [CrossRef]
33. Adedayo, A.M.; Olafiranye, O.; Smith, D.; Hill, A.; Zizi, F.; Brown, C.; Jean-Louis, G. Obstructive sleep apnea and dyslipidemia: Evidence and underlying mechanism. *Sleep Breath.* **2014**, *18*, 13–18. [CrossRef]
34. Gündüz, C.; Basoglu, O.K.; Hedner, J.; Zou, D.; Bonsignore, M.R.; Hein, H.; Staats, R.; Pataka, A.; Barbe, F.; Sliwinski, P. Obstructive sleep apnoea independently predicts lipid levels: Data from the European sleep apnea database. *Respirology* **2018**, *23*, 1180–1189. [CrossRef]
35. Kang, H.H.; Kang, J.Y.; Ha, J.H.; Lee, J.; Kim, S.K.; Moon, H.S.; Lee, S.H. The associations between anthropometric indices and obstructive sleep apnea in a Korean population. *PLoS ONE* **2014**, *9*, e114463. [CrossRef]
36. Soylu, A.C.; Levent, E.; Sarıman, N.; Yurtlu, Ş.; Alparslan, S.; Saygı, A. Obstructive sleep apnea syndrome and anthropometric obesity indexes. *Sleep Breath.* **2012**, *16*, 1151–1158. [CrossRef]
37. Subramanian, S.; Jayaraman, G.; Majid, H.; Aguilar, R.; Surani, S. Influence of gender and anthropometric measures on severity of obstructive sleep apnea. *Sleep Breath.* **2012**, *16*, 1091–1095. [CrossRef]
38. Arokiasamy, P. India's escalating burden of non-communicable diseases. *Lancet Glob. Health* **2018**, *6*, e1262–e1263. [CrossRef]

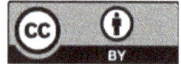

© 2019 by the authors. Licensee MDPI, Basel, Switzerland. This article is an open access article distributed under the terms and conditions of the Creative Commons Attribution (CC BY) license (http://creativecommons.org/licenses/by/4.0/).

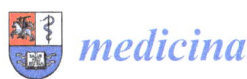

Review

Exhaled Breath Analysis in Obstructive Sleep Apnea Syndrome: A Review of the Literature

Panaiotis Finamore [1], Simone Scarlata [1,*], Vittorio Cardaci [2] and Raffaele Antonelli Incalzi [1]

1. Unit of Geriatrics, Campus Bio-Medico di Roma University, via Alvaro del Portillo 200, 00128 Rome, Italy
2. Pulmonary Rehabilitation, IRCCS San Raffaele Pisana, 00166 Rome, Italy
* Correspondence: s.scarlata@unicampus.it; Tel.: +39-06-22-541-1167; Fax: +39-06-22-541-456

Received: 27 June 2019; Accepted: 22 August 2019; Published: 27 August 2019

Abstract: *Background and Objectives:* Obstructive sleep apnea syndrome (OSAS) represents an independent risk factor for cardiovascular, metabolic and neurological events. Polysomnography is the gold-standard for the diagnosis, however is expensive and time-consuming and not suitable for widespread use. Breath analysis is an innovative, non-invasive technique, able to provide clinically relevant information about OSAS. This systematic review was aimed to outline available evidence on the role of exhaled breath analysis in OSAS, taking into account the techniques' level of adherence to the recently proposed technical standards. *Materials and Methods:* Articles reporting original data on exhaled breath analysis in OSAS were identified through a computerized and manual literature search and screened. Duplicate publications, case reports, case series, conference papers, expert opinions, comments, reviews and meta-analysis were excluded. *Results:* Fractional exhaled Nitric Oxide (FeNO) is higher in OSAS patients than controls, however its absolute value is within reported normal ranges. FeNO association with AHI is controversial, as well as its change after continuous positive airway pressure (C-PAP) therapy. Exhaled breath condensate (EBC) is acid in OSAS, cytokines and oxidative stress markers are elevated, they positively correlate with AHI and normalize after treatment. The analysis of volatile organic compounds (VOCs) by spectrometry or electronic nose is able to discriminate OSAS from healthy controls. The main technical issues regards the dilution of EBC and the lack of external validation in VOCs studies. *Conclusions:* Exhaled breath analysis has a promising role in the understanding of mechanisms underpinning OSAS and has demonstrated a clinical relevance in identifying individuals affected by the disease, in assessing the response to treatment and, potentially, to monitor patient's adherence to mechanical ventilation. Albeit the majority of the technical standards proposed by the ERS committee have been followed by existing papers, further work is needed to uniform the methodology.

Keywords: obstructive sleep apnea; inflammation; FeNO; exhaled breath condensate; volatile organic compounds

1. Introduction

Obstructive sleep apnea syndrome (OSAS) is a highly prevalent sleep breathing disorder characterized by intermittent reduction (hypopnea) and/or cessation (apnea) of airflow due to upper airways collapse and represents an independent risk factor for cardiovascular [1,2], metabolic [3], neurological diseases [4,5], and motor vehicle accidents [6]. The disease is also common in children, with a prevalence of 1–4%, and associates with behavioral and cognitive deficits [7,8]. The exact mechanism underpinning these detrimental effects is still unknown, however the pro-inflammatory state and the oxidative stress likely due to the intermittent hypoxia are deemed to play a key role [9]; indeed, the use of a continue positive airways pressure ventilation (C-PAP) has demonstrated to be effective in reducing the airways collapse, minimizing the endothelial stress and, consequently, the pro-inflammatory state [10]. Given the severity of the complications, a correct diagnosis is warranted and the gold-standard is represented by polysomnography (PSG) [11] that, however requires specialized personnel and devoted setting which limits a wide use of the tool and compels to screen the population to refer to the specialist. Questionnaires are validated screening tools, however up to 45% of patients referred with the suspicion of OSAS are not confirmed by PSG [11,12], thus new approaches in identifying patients affected by OSAS need to be identified.

Exhaled breath is abundant in volatile organic compounds (VOCs), part of which are endogenous and produced by cellular metabolism. Exhaled breath analysis, proved to detect the metabolic changes induced by OSAS, can be applied as a non-invasive tool able to shed light on the pathways modified by the disease, and also to provide a more rapid and economic instrument for diagnosis, monitoring and, eventually, characterization of the disease. Systematic reviews in this field of research are already available in literature [13,14], but, recently, several studies have been published that have enriched the available amount of evidence; furthermore, all the available reviews preceded the recently published European Respiratory Society (ERS) statement about the technical standards to follow in the exhaled breath analysis published in 2017 [15] and is therefore unclear, at the moment, to which extent the previous works adhered such methodological standards.

The aim of this systematic review is therefore to outline the newly available evidences on the exhaled breath analysis role in OSAS, taking into account whether they conform to the proposed ERS technical standards.

2. Materials and Methods

We performed a computerized and manual literature search on PubMed, limited to English language articles published up to May 2019, to identify articles reporting original data on exhaled breath analysis in obstructive sleep apnea. We entered the following MeSH terms: Obstructive Sleep Apnea; Obstructive Sleep Apneas Syndrome; OSA; OSAS; in combination with: volatile organic compounds; VOC; electronic nose; gas chromatography mass spectrometry; spectrometry; exhaled breath condensate; EBC; nitric oxide; FeNO. Two authors (P.F. and S.S.) performed the literature search and assessed the eligibility of identified publications independently. All studies that evaluated exhaled breath analysis in OSAS were screened. Duplicate publications, case reports, case series, conference papers, expert opinions, comments, reviews and meta-analysis were excluded. The selection process is summarized in Figure 1. The literature search has been integrated with other relevant studies about methodological and clinical issues.

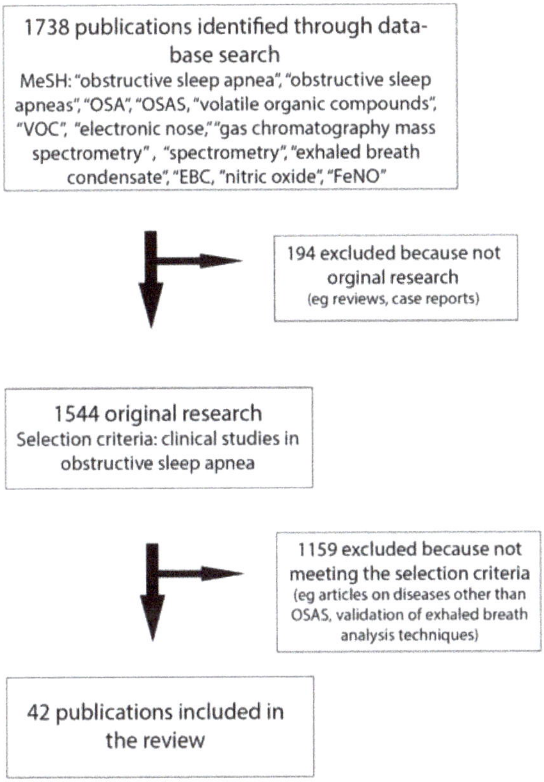

```
┌─────────────────────────────────────────┐
│ 1738 publications identified through    │
│ database search                         │
│ MeSH: "obstructive sleep apnea",        │
│ "obstructive sleep apneas", "OSA",      │
│ "OSAS", "volatile organic compounds",   │
│ "VOC", "electronic nose", "gas          │
│ chromatography mass spectrometry",      │
│ "spectrometry", "exhaled breath         │
│ condensate", "EBC", "nitric oxide",     │
│ "FeNO"                                  │
└─────────────────────────────────────────┘
                    │
                    ├──▶ 194 excluded because not
                    │    original research
                    │    (eg reviews, case reports)
                    ▼
┌─────────────────────────────────────────┐
│ 1544 original research                  │
│ Selection criteria: clinical studies in │
│ obstructive sleep apnea                 │
└─────────────────────────────────────────┘
                    │
                    ├──▶ 1159 excluded because not
                    │    meeting the selection criteria
                    │    (eg articles on diseases other than
                    │    OSAS, validation of exhaled breath
                    │    analysis techniques)
                    ▼
┌─────────────────────────────────────────┐
│ 42 publications included in             │
│ the review                              │
└─────────────────────────────────────────┘
```

Figure 1. PRISMA diagram showing the flow of information through the different phases of the reviewing process.

3. Results

The thirty-six studies included in the review encompass the three main domains of exhaled breath analysis: the fractional exhaled nitric oxide (FeNO), the exhaled breath condensate (EBC) and the exhaled VOCs. The characteristics of the main studies included in the review are summarized in Tables 1–3.

3.1. FeNO and Exhaled Carbon Monoxide (eCO)

Nitric oxide (NO) is a gaseous molecule produced by nitric oxide synthase (NOS) enzymes from L-arginine and oxygen. There are three isoforms of NOS, two are constitutively produced (endothelial NOS–eNOS– and neuronal NOS–nNOS–) and one is inducible (iNOS), increasing during inflammation [16], as that characterizing airways in asthmatic patients. Indeed, the FeNO in the gas phase emerged in the last decade of the last century as an innovative diagnostic marker of asthma [17,18]. Being non-invasive and easy to perform, FeNO raised a wide interest, allowing a deeper understanding of mechanisms underpinning its production and addressing technical issues related its measurement. Nowadays, FeNO is considered a marker of T-helper 2 cell-type inflammation, rather than a marker of asthma per se, and a marker of response to corticosteroid treatment in those patients [19].

The study of FeNO in the diagnosis of OSAS has led to contradictory findings. Indeed, while some studies described a raising of FeNO level in OSAS [20–25], the majority did not confirm the finding [26–30] or just showed a higher concentration in OSAS patients when compared with non-obese healthy controls [31–33]. Besides, even considering only those studies with a positive finding, the FeNO level, albeit statistically higher than healthy controls, did not reach a clinical significance. Indeed, in all studies the mean FeNO expressed in part per billion (ppb) was below 30 ppb, which means that OSAS patients are classified in the group of individuals without airway inflammation (or without eosinophilic inflammation) or in the grey zone between 25 and 50 ppb according to the ATS guidelines [19], the same groups of healthy controls. One possible explanation of the low level of FeNO despite the inflammatory state can be the different location of the process, closer to the alveoli than the airways or in the opposite, as the result of a topical, mechanically induced inflammation at the level of the upper airway caused by snoring and apnea associated mechanical stress [34,35]. Indeed, international guidelines suggest to use a flow of 50 mL/s for the measurement of FeNO, however it is not high enough to allow the collection of the alveolar portion of NO [36]. Albeit some studies have found a statistically significant higher concentration of exhaled nitric oxide (eNO) at a flow of 250 mL/s or more in association with an elevated concentration of NO in the gas phase of Alveoli (CaNO) [22,25,37], Fortuna and colleagues reported a lower CaNO in OSAS patients than healthy controls [23] and Foresi and colleagues did not find a difference in CaNO between normotensive OSAS patients and controls [30]. The more validated hypothesis is that the increased inflammation damages the alveolar endothelium reducing the expression of the eNOS and the diffusion of NO [38]. Mechanisms of inflammation induced by OSAS are reproduced in Figure 2.

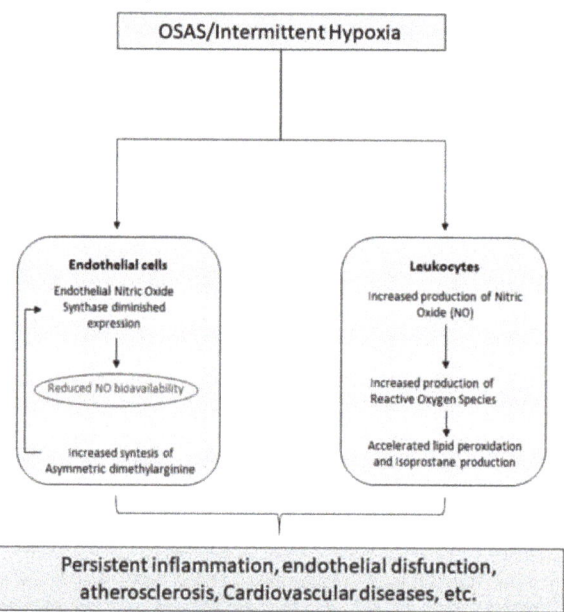

Figure 2. Principal inflammatory pathways induced by OSAS.

Furthermore, it is still unclear whether an overnight change in the production of eNO exists or not. While some studies reported an overnight increase in FeNO [20,24] and in the concentration of nitric oxide exhaled by the nose (nasal nitric oxide–nNO–) and by the mouth (orale nitrix oxide–oNO–) [39] in OSAS patients [20,39], other studies failed to confirm the evidence [21], or they found an overnight increase limited to subgroups of OSAS, such as obese OSAS patients [29] or children with mild OSAS but not moderate/severe [28], or healthy controls [39].

Finally, eNO has been proposed as a marker to monitor the efficacy of C-PAP therapy. Indeed, evidence in literature suggests that one-to-three month C-PAP treatment is effective in reducing FeNO [22–24] and increasing CaNO [23]. The effect should also be time-dependent, at least for

FeNO, since a single or 2-nigth treatment with C-PAP increases CaNO [30,40] but do not reduce FeNO [30]. This suggest that C-PAP, normalizing oxygen saturation, reduces inflammation and oxidative stress, promoting alveolar endothelial function and therefore candidates CaNO as a marker of endothelial function.

Even the association of the eNO with the apnea-hypopnea index (AHI) is controversial. Indeed, while some studies found a strong and positive correlation between FeNO and AHI, with a r of 0.8–0.9 [23,33], or oNO and AHI (r: 0.46) [32] and a negative one between CaNO and AHI, with a r of 0.9 [23], this was not confirmed by other studies [20–22,27,28,39,41].

Knowledge about exhaled carbon monoxide (eCO) in OSAS is more limited than FeNO. To the extent possible, eCO has been reported higher only in severe OSAS [42], it has a weak correlation with AHI [42] and it is not normalized after one-month of C-PAP [22], probably because it needs a longer period to be normalized.

3.2. Exhaled Breath Condensate

The alveolar and airway lining fluids (ALF) contain hydrophobic and hydrophilic nonvolatile and volatile compounds which are continuously released into the environment as droplets created during breathing. In contrast to bronchoalveolar lavage, EBC is a noninvasive way to sample these compounds by directing the exhaled breath through a cooling device. The sample, mostly composed by water vapour, can be stored or immediately analyzed. Albeit noninvasive, EBC composition is highly influenced by the collection and the condenser procedure, which undermine the reliability of the achieved results. Principles of functioning of exhaled breath condensate technology is summarized in Figure 3.

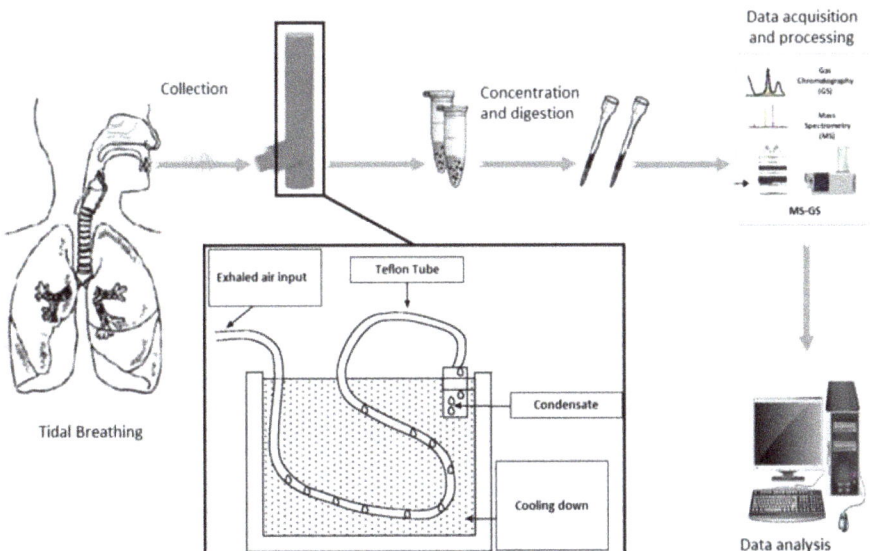

Figure 3. Principles of functioning of exhaled breath condensate technology.

3.2.1. EBC pH

Given the inflammatory and pro-inflammatory state characterizing OSAS, EBC pH in OSAS was expected to be lower than healthy controls. The hypothesis has been confirmed by all the studies carried out so far, with the exception of that by Greulich and colleagues [43], with a mean absolute value of EBC pH in OSAS around 7.4, by far below the first quartile of EBC pH distribution in healthy subjects and equal to the fifth percentile [44]. pH has shown a negative correlation with AHI (r: −0.66), sleep time with a SaO_2 < 90% (r: −0.62) and neck circumference (r: −0.63) [31], but also with body-mass index (BMI) (r: −0.54). Although Petrosyan and colleagues demonstrated that OSAS EBC pH is lower than controls, even if obese [22], the finding has not been confirmed by Carpagnano et al. [31], raising doubts about the association between EBC acidity and OSAS. Albeit it is not possible to exclude that obesity, rather than OSAS, reduces EBC pH, probably by increasing the likelihood to have gastro-esophageal reflux, it seems that EBC acidity is due to OSAS. Indeed, after the treatment with C-PAP EBC pH increases [22], becoming closer to normal reference values. A change of the EBC pH after C-PAP or surgical treatment has not been confirmed by other studies [43,45], however in both cases the EBC pH value of OSAS patients was already normal at baseline. No significant difference has been found between OSA smokers and non-smokers [46]. To conclude, all studies analyzing EBC pH performed de-aeration before the analysis, but did not performed the analysis in real time or immediately after collection without freezing or storing EBC, as suggested by international guidelines [15]. OSAS seems to increase EBC acidity, however exist a variability in the EBC pH that compels to investigate the effect of other factors.

3.2.2. EBC Cytokines

EBC cytokine level has been studied in OSAS patients. As expected, all studies confirmed that the concentration of IL-6, TNF-α, IL-8 and ICAM-1 is higher than healthy controls, while IL-10 concentration, which has anti-inflammatory properties, is lower [46–49]. However, there is a wide range of cytokine concentrations among the studies: indeed, while the mean EBC IL-6 concentration was in the order of decades of pg/mL in some studies [47,48], it was below the unit in other studies [46,50], notwithstanding the concentration was expressed in the same unit of measurement. Similarly, the concentration of TNF-α in the studies of Li and colleagues [48,51] was ten times the concentration of TNF-α in the study of Antonopoulou and colleagues [46]. Hence, even pro-inflammatory cytokines seem elevated in OSAS and anti-inflammatory cytokines reduced, sampling procedure should be revised, because confounding factors, as dilution, seem to have affected the absolute value. Other confounding factors to take into account are obesity and smoking. Indeed, while some studies do not report a difference in IL-6 level between smoking and non-smoking OSAS patients [46], other studies suggest a pro-inflammatory effect of smoking [48]. Noteworthy, no doubts are on the pro-inflammatory role of obesity, with all studies confirming an elevated concentration of EBC IL-6, IL-8 and ICAM-1 in obese than normal weight individuals [47,49]. Being inflammation in OSAS closely related with intermittent hypoxia, it is not surprising that AHI was positively correlated with EBC IL-6 (r: 0.6–0.8) [47,48], ICAM-1 (r: 0.7) [49] and TNF-α (r: 0.85) [48] and negatively correlated with EBC IL-10 (r: −0.63) [51]. As expected, EBC IL-6 also positively correlated with the neck circumference (r: 0.5) [47]. EBC cytokines are stable over time if patients do not start a treatment [51], while effective treatment reduces their concentration. Indeed, even with different absolute values, two studies demonstrating the effectiveness of C-PAP therapy [50,51], but also the positive role of oral appliances and surgery in abating inflammation and thus EBC cytokine concentration [51].

3.2.3. EBC Oxidative Stress

The EBC concentration of 8-isoprostane, a product of the lipid peroxidation of arachidonic acid and marker of oxidative stress, has been repeatedly found elevated in adult patients affected by OSAS [22,46–48,52,53], and in children [28]. The mean value in OSAS patients is heterogeneous, ranging from 6 to more than 30 pg/mL, and overlaps with the mean values observed in healthy controls [46,48]. Smoking seems to affect the marker concentration [48], while the role of obesity is conflicting. Indeed, while Petrosyan and colleagues found a higher level of 8-isoprostane in healthy non obese than obese individuals, both were significantly lower than OSAS patients [22], Carpagnano and colleagues observed exactly the opposite, also failing to discriminate OSAS from obese controls by 8-isoprostane concentration [47]. 8-isoprostane has shown a positive correlation with AHI, with a r of 0.4–0.5, [22,28,46–48,52,53] and neck circumference (r: 0.5–0.6) [47,52]. Interestingly, the concentration of 8-isoprostane is higher in the morning than in the evening in OSAS patients, with the latter similar to the concentration of healthy controls [52]. C-PAP therapy is effective in reducing the concentration of 8-isoprostane, but it is also reduced by oral appliances and surgery [50–52].

More limited evidence exists on the EBC concentration of hydrogen peroxide (H_2O_2). To the extent possible, H_2O_2 seems elevated in OSAS [22,54], regardless of patient's BMI [22]. Noteworthy, obesity is associated with an increase in the H_2O_2 concentration in healthy controls [22]. H_2O_2 is also positively associated with the AHI, with the same correlation of 8-isoprostante [22], and thus with the severity of the disease, being higher in patients with moderate to severe than mild OSAS [54]. This marker is not modified by one month of C-PAP therapy [22]. While Petrosyan and colleagues clearly recommended the use of a filter on the inspiratory valve to avoid an environmental conditioning [22], it is not clear whether Malakasoti and colleagues did the same [54]. Both studies did not perform the measurement of H_2O_2 immediately after the collection, as suggested by the ERS guidelines [15].

3.2.4. Other EBC Markers

Other markers assessed in the EBC of OSAS patients are: urates, leukotrienes and leptin. EBC concentration of acid uric, which has antioxidant capacity, has been studied in children and resulted significantly higher than healthy controls [55], probably having a role in contrasting the increased oxidative stress driven by the disease. Similarly, leukotrienes (leukotriene B4, which is also associated with the severity of the disease [22,56] and leukotriene C4/D4/E4), lipid mediators prompting inflammation, are elevated in OSAS, even though with a completely different absolute value in pg/mL among studies. Indeed, the concentration found in one study in OSAS patients completely overlaps with that found in healthy controls in another study [22,56]. Contrary to the expectations, prostaglandins (PGE2) did not show any difference between children affected by OSAS and controls [56]. Furthermore, no role seems to have leptin as an EBC biomarker of OSAS. Indeed, while obese OSAS patients have higher concentration than controls, non-obese OSAS and obese controls have the same concentration, suggesting, together with a strong and positive correlation with BMI, that obesity rather than OSAS affects the concentration of this mediator [57].

3.3. Volatile Organic Compounds: Spectrometry and Electronic Nose

Exhaled breath is abundant in VOCs with very low concentration, most of which are undetectable by the human nose. These molecules in part originate from the endogenous metabolism and human gut and airway microbiome [58], thus their study might provide information about any diseases threatening the internal homeostasis and thus help address their diagnosis, disease severity stratification and prognosis, as already demonstrated in other respiratory diseases [59]. To date, there exist two main approaches to the study of VOCs: the first aims to identify single biomarkers related to the disease in the mixture of molecules and it is based on the use of spectrometry, often coupled with separation techniques as gas-chromatography; the second is aimed to identify a pattern in the mixture able to discriminate, through the use of a pattern-recognition approach, the disease from other conditions and it is based on the use of electronic-noses. Both have been applied in the study of OSAS, either alone or in association.

The use of analytical techniques have demonstrated a good accuracy in discriminating OSAS patients from healthy controls [60], even if obese [61]. However, no study has so far identified a single molecule able to discriminate OSAS from controls, thus discrimination is based on a set of VOCs. Greulich and colleagues reported in their study an increase in OSAS of 2-methylfuran, 2-(methylthio)-ethanol and hexanal and a reduction in 3-methylbutanal or 3-methylbutyraldehyde and acetone [60]. Interestingly, an increase in 2-methylfuran in serum and pharyngeal wash of those patients was also reported. However, none of the compounds described by Greulich were also identified by Dragonieri and colleagues, who reported a good discriminative capacity between OSAS and obese controls basing on the following compounds: tetrachloroethene, 2,3,5-trimethylhexane, β-pinene, 1,3,5-trimethylbenzene, 9-methylacridine, tetradecane, 6,10-dimethyl-5,9-undecadien-2-one and β-ionone [61]. Besides, Aoki and colleagues found that although almost all the aromatic and satured hydrocarbons are more expressed in the exhaled breath of severe OSAS patients, only isoprene is always elevated in OSAS, regardless the severity of the disease [62].

A good discriminative accuracy in discriminating OSAS from normal weight controls and chronic obstructive pulmonary disease (COPD) patients has also been demonstrated by the use of electronic noses, which showed a lower accuracy in discriminating people affected by the disease from healthy obese controls [43,63–65]. As already observed for other exhaled breath markers (e.g., 8-isoprostane), the breath pattern changed overnight in OSAS patients but not in controls, likely due to the inflammation and oxidative stress promoted by the intermittent hypoxia; indeed there was a difference in breath pattern between OSAS and controls only in the morning. Noteworthy, the difference is still present after the exclusion of patients suffering from gastro-esophageal reflux and COPD [66]. The finding is in line with that of Olopade and colleagues who reported a higher concentration of oral pentane in the morning than in the evening [39]. While some studies found a positive correlation between the breath pattern and the AHI [43], other studies failed to confirm the finding [66]. Albeit apparently contradictory, it is possible that the association between AHI and breath pattern is mediated by patients' comorbidities, as suggested by Incalzi and colleagues [67]. Breath-pattern is sensitive to the effects of the C-PAP therapy, indeed concentrations of isoprene and acetone decrease [62] and it is possible to discriminate treated and untreated patients with good accuracy [68]; even a single night treatment is associated with a change in the breath pattern. Interestingly, the breath pattern change does not have the same characteristics in all OSAS patients, with two different types of response being distinguished depending on the comorbidities of those individuals [67]. Noteworthily, almost all the studies did not perform an external validation of the discriminative model, hence it is not possible to exclude an overfitting of the models, even though minimized by the use of internal cross-validation. Technical and operative descriptions of these approaches have been summarized in Figure 4 and discussed in detail elsewhere [69,70].

Table 1. Exhaled nitric oxide for the diagnosis of OSAS patients.

First Author (Year) [Reference]	OSAS	AHI	NO	Device	FeNO ppb	HC	NO ppb	p-Value
Zhang (2018) [20]	75	28.1 e/h	FeNO (1) nNO (2)	NIOX MINO® 50 mL/s	(1) 21.08 (8.79) (2) 487 (115.8)	30	(1) 16.9 (6.86) (2) 413 (73.1)	0.02
Przybylowski (2006) [21]	66	40.3 e/h	FeNO	CA 45–55	23.1 (14.8)	53	16.8 (9.8)	<0.05
Petrosyan (2008) [22]	26	63.7 e/h	FeNO (1) nNO (2) eCO (3)	LR2000 CA 250 mL/s	(1) 7.1 (4.6) (2) 610 (222) (3) 6.4 (2.9)	9 O * 10 NO †	(1) 5 (1.1) * (1) 4.2 (1.9) (2) 366 (169) * (2) 539 (264) † (3) 4.8 (1) * (3) 4.7 (1.2) †	<0.05 <0.05 <0.01 NS <0.05 <0.05
Olopade (1997) [39]	16	47.7 e/h	FeNO (1) nNO	CA NA	(1) 6.6 (0.8)	8	(1) 6.8 (1.3)	NA
JalilMirmohammadi (2014) [29]	31 O * 16 NO †	39.5 e/h 40.1 e/h	FeNO	NObreath® 50 mL/s	14.1, 3–31 * 15.8, 2–31 †	7	22.1, 5–58	NS
Gut (2016) [41]	28	6.6 e/h	nNO	Eco Medics AG	867 (371)	23	644 (166)	0.047
Fortuna (2011) [23]	30	NA >15 e/h	FeNO (1) CaNO (2)	NIOX 50 mL/s	(1) 27.2 (18)	30	(1) 16.7 (8)	0.0006
Foresi (2007) [30]	34	31.3 e/h	FeNO	NOA 280 50,120,190, 250 e 300 mL/s	21.8 (1.9)	9	15.4 (1.7)	NS
Duarte (2019) [26]	199	30.1 e/h	FeNO	NIOX MINO® 50 mL/s	20.2 (14.5)	30	16.9 (10.6)	0.221
Depalo (2008) [33]	18 O	59.1 e/h	FeNO (1) iNOS (2)	CA 45 mL/s	(1) 23.1 (2.1)	15 O * 10 NO †	(1) 17.9 (2.1) * (1) 7.2 (0.6) †	NS <0.001
Culla (2010) [32]	39	NA >10 e/h	FeNO (1) oNO (2)	CA 50 mL/s	(1) 23.1, 19–28 (2) 104, 80–135	26 AS * 15 CR † 24 ‡	(1) 40, 32–50 * (1) 22, 16–32 † (1) 11, 8–14 ‡ (2) 71, 56–91 * (2) 54, 40–73 † (2) 63, 59–73 ‡	NS NS <0.001 0.015 0.009 <0.001
Carpagnano (2008) [31]	30 O	59.1 e/h	FeNO	CA 45 mL/s	31.6 (1.6)	20 O * 10 NO †	27.1 (1.8) * 4.8 (0.7) †	NS <0.001

Table 1. Cont.

First Author (Year) [Reference]	OSAS	AHI	Molecule	NO	Device	FeNO ppb	HC	NO ppb	p-Value
Duong-Quoy (2015) [25]	52	25.6 e/h		FeNO (1) CaNO (2)	FeNO+ 50,100,150,350 mL/s	(1) 16.7 (11.4) (2) 4 (1.7)	30	(1) 9.4 (6.6) (2) 2.2 (0.7)	0.003 0.001
Barreto (2018) [28]	17 CH mild * 17 CH mod/sev †	2.3 e/h 8.6 e/h		FeNO	HyPair FENO 50 mL/s	11, 7.9–14.8 * 10, 6.5–16 †	20	13.5, 8.7–19.9	NS
Agusti (1999) [27]	24	55 e/h		FeNO	CA NA	22.2 (3)	7	19.7 (3.2)	NS
Chua (2013) [24]	75	40 e/h		FeNO	NIOX MINO® 50 mL/s	13.4 (6.5)	29	6.5 (3.5)	<0.001

For those studies analyzing the change of FeNO during the night, the mean (SD) is that before the night. Legend: OSAS: obstructive sleep apnea syndrome; AHI: apnea-hypopnea index (e/h: events per hour); HC: healthy controls; FeNO: fractional exhaled nitric oxide; nNO: nasal nitric oxide; oNO: oral nitric oxide; O: obese; NO: not obese; CA: chemiluminescence analyser; AS: asthma; CR: chronic rhinitis/rhinosinusitis. Symbols (*,†,‡) are used to link the value with the subgroup.

Table 2. Exhaled breath condensate for the diagnosis of OSAS.

First Author (Year) [Reference]	OSAS	AHI	Molecule	Standards	Value	HC	Value	p-Value
Carpagnano (2008) [31]	30 OS	59.1 e/h	pH	Volume collection ✗ Tidal breathing ✓ Nose clip ✓ Storage ✓ Deaeration ✓	7.48 (0.07)	20 ON * 10 NO †	7.68 (0.08) * 7.99 (0.03) †	NS <0.01
Carpagnano (2003) [52]	18	59.2 e/h	8-Isoprost.	Volume collection ✓ Tidal breathing ✓ Nose clip ✓ Storage ✓	9.5 (1.9) pg/mL	12	6.7 (0.2) pg/mL	<0.001
Petrosyan (2008) [22]	26	63.7 e/h	pH (1) 8-Isoprost.(2) Leuk.B4 (3) H2O2 (4)	Volume collection ✓ Tidal breathing ✓ Nose clip ✓ Deaeration ✓ Storage ✓	(1) 7.2 (0.69) (2) 12 (6) pg/mL (3) 8 (6) pg/mL (4) 5.8 (8.9) uM	9 O * 10NO †	(1) 7.79 (0.09) * (1) 7.77 (0.05) † (2) 4 (0.2) pg/mL * (2) 5 (1.9) pg/mL † (3) NA * (3) NA † (4) 1.2 (0.9) uM * (4) 0.3 (0.4) uM †	<0.01 <0.01 <0.001 <0.001 <0.001 <0.001 <0.05 <0.01

Table 2. Cont.

First Author (Year) [Reference]	OSAS	AHI	Molecule	Standards	Value	HC	Value	p-Value
Vlasic (2011) ▲ [55]	17	3.54 e/h	Urates	Volume collection ✔ Tidal breathing ✔ Nose clip ✘ Storage ✘	86, 28–113 µmol/L	12	31, 23–42 µmol/L	0.046
Malakasioti (2012) ▲ [54]	12 Mo-S (1) 22 Mild (2)	13.6 e/h 2.8 e/h	log(H2O2)	Volume collection ✔ Tidal breathing ✔ Nose clip ✔ Storage ✔	0.4 (1.1) −0.9 (1.3)	16	−1.2 (1.2)	(1vs3) 0.003 (1vs2) 0.015
Li (2009) [48]	22 Mild * 22 Mo † 24 S ‡	14.1 e/h 29.7 e/h 70.1 e/h	8-Isoprost.(1) IL-6 (2) TNF-α (3) IL-10 (4)		(1) 15.5 (2) pg/mL * (1) 18.8 (2) pg/mL † (1) 21.8 (2) pg/mL ‡ (2) 8.4 (1) pg/mL * (2) 13.9 (2) pg/mL † (2) 15.5 (2) pg/mL ‡ (3) 96.1 (8) pg/mL * (3) 116 (11) pg/mL † (3) 128.2 (8) pg/mL ‡ (4) 48.2 (6) pg/mL * (4) 31.2 (5) pg/mL † (4) 24 (4) pg/mL ‡	22 HNS ⨍ 10 HS ‖	(1) 12.6 (2) pg/mL ⨍ (1) 16.8 (2) pg/mL ‖ (2) 6.8 (1) pg/mL ⨍ (2) 10.9 (2) pg/mL ‖ (3) 83.7 (4) pg/mL ⨍ (3) 97 (6) pg/mL ‖ (4) 56.8 (7) pg/mL ⨍ (4) 38.6 (7) pg/mL ‖	(1) <0.001 (2) <0.001 (3) <0.001 (4) <0.001
Carpagnano (2002) [47]	18	59.2 e/h	8-Isoprost.(1) IL-6 (2)	Volume collection ✘ Tidal breathing ✔ Nose clip ✘ Storage ✔	(1) 7.4 (0.7) pg/mL (2) 8.7 (0.3) pg/mL	10 ON * 15 NO †	(1) 5 (0.3) pg/mL * (1) 4.5 (1) pg/mL † (2) 2.1(0.2) pg/m *1 (2) 1.6(0.1) pg/mL †	0.4 <0.005 <0.05 <0.001
Goldbart (2006) ▲ [56]	29 Mild * 21 Mo-S †	< 5 e/h > 5 e/h	Leuk.B4 (1) LeukTC4/D4/E4 (2) PGE2 (3)	Volume collection ✘ Tidal breathing ✔ Nose clip ✘ Storage ✔	(1) 66.4 (4) pg/mL * (1) 97.6 (6) pg/mL † (2) 27.6 (8) pg/mL * (2) 45.1 (11) pg/mL † (3) ≈ 29 pg/mL * (3) ≈ 35 pg/mL †	NA	(1) 27.8 (4) pg/mL (2) 15.7 (8) pg/mL (3) ≈ 19 pg/mL	<0.001 <0.001 NS
Carpagnano (S 2010) [57]	36 OS * 28 NOS †	57.6 e/h 40.8 e/h	Leptin	Volume collection ✘ Tidal breathing ✔ Nose clip ✔ Storage ✔	5.12, 3.8–6.6 ng/mL ‡ 4.1, 3.9–5.2 ng/mL †	24 ON ‡ 20 NO ⨍	4.2, 3.6–5 ng/mL ‡ 3.2, 2.4–4 ng/mL ⨍	<0.05

Table 2. Cont.

First Author (Year) [Reference]	OSAS	AHI	Molecule	Standards	Value	HC	Value	p-Value
Barreto (2018) ▲ [28]	17 CH mild * 17 CH Mo-S †	2.3 e/h 8.6 e/h	8-Isoprost.	Volume collection ✗ Tidal breathing ✔ Nose clip ✔ Storage ✔	45, 30–88 pg/mL * 52, 39–130 pg/mL †	20	19.2, 12–32 pg/mL	<0.01 <0.01
Antonopoulou (2008) [46]	45	39 e/h	pH (1) 8-Isoprost. (2) IL-6 (3) TNF-α (4)	Volume collection ✗ Tidal breathing ✔ Nose clip? Storage ✔ Deaeration ?	(1) 7.44 (0.2) (2) 30.5 (19) pg/mL (3) 0.53 (0.3) pg/mL (4) 1.4 (0.9) pg/mL	25	(1) 7.46 (0.1) (2) 12 (3) pg/mL (3) 0.21 (0) pg/mL (4) 0.6 (0.3) pg/mL	0.0009 <0.0001 0.03 0.0002
Carpagnano (J 2010) [49]	12 OS * 10 NO †	48.8 e/h	IL-8 (1) ICAM-1 (2)	Volume collection ✗ Tidal breathing ✔ Nose clip ✔ Storage ✔	(1) 17.5 (2) pg/mL * (1) 14.8 (1.9) pg/mL † (2) 100 (3.6) pg/mL * (2) 88.6 (3.9) pg/mL †	10 ON 8 NO	(1) 17 (0.7) pg/mL * (1) 7 (0.5) pg/mL † (2) 93 (2.6) pg/mL * (2) 51 (1.2) pg/mL †	NS <0.001 NS <0.001
Karamanli (2014) [50]	35 C-PAP	3.8 vs. 45.6	8-Isoprost. (1) IL-6 (2) TNF-α (3) Peroxynitr. (4)	Volume collection ✗ Tidal breathing ✔ Nose clip ✔ Storage ✔	(1) 3 vs. 5.7 pg/mL (2) 0.3 vs. 1.1 pg/mL (3) 26.8 vs. 29 pg/mL (4) 4.6 vs. 17.3 pg/mL	-	-	0.027 <0.001 <0.001 0.037
Li (2008) [51]	33 C-PAP† 28 UNT ‡ 2 OrAp * 5 SURG ≠ 22 HC	24.7 vs. 45.7 32.5 vs. 31.4 12.9 vs. 38.6 28.8 vs. 32.7	8-Isoprost. (1) IL-6 (2) TNF-α (3) IL-10 (4)	Volume collection ✗ Tidal breathing ✔ Nose clip ✔ Storage ✔	(1) 15 vs. 20 pg/mL † (1) 17 vs. 17 pg/mL ‡(1) 12 vs. 18 pg/mL * (1) 13 vs. 20 pg/mL ≠ (2) 10 vs. 14 pg/mL † (2) 11 vs. 11 pg/mL ‡ (2) 8 vs. 11 pg/mL * (2) 9 vs. 13 pg/mL ≠		(3) 97 vs. 118 pg/mL † (3) 108 vs. 108 pg/mL ‡ (3) 105 vs. 119 pg/mL * (3) 88 vs. 117 pg/mL ≠ (4) 42 vs. 21 pg/mL † (4) 38 vs. 38 pg/mL ‡ (4) 37 vs. 35 pg/mL * (4) 50 vs. 31 pg/mL ≠	Unknown

▲ Study carried out in children. Legend: OSAS: obstructive sleep apnea syndrome; AHI: apnea-hypopnea index (e/h: events per hour); HC: healthy controls; Mild: Mo-S: moderate-severe; OS: obese OSAS; NOS: non-obese OSAS; ON: obese healthy controls; NO: non-obese healthy controls; C-PAP: continuous positive airway pressure; UNT: untreated; OrAp: oral appliances; SURG: surgery. ✔: technical standard satisfied; ✗: technical standard not satisfied. Symbols (*, †, ‡, ≠) are used to link the value with the subgroup.

Table 3. Volatile organic compounds analysis for the diagnosis of OSAS patients.

First Author (Year) [Reference]	OSAS	AHI	Device	Standards	Controls	Discriminative capacity	p-Value
Greulich (2013) [43]	40	33.6 e/h	E-nose (Cyranose320) Disposable bags	Internal cross-validation ✓ External validation set ✓	20	AUROC 0.85 (95%CI 0.74–0.96)	-
Dragonieri (2016) [65]	13 (6 validation set)	44.8 e/h	E-nose (Cyranose320) Disposable bags	Internal cross-validation ✓ External validation set ✓	15 COPD (6 validation set) 13 OVS (6 validation set)	AUROC OSAS vs. OVS.: 1 AUROC OSAS vs. COPD: 0.83	<0.001 <0.01
Kunos (2015) [66]	17 OSAS 9 habitual snorers	29.8 e/h	E-nose Mylar bags	Internal cross-validation ✓ External validation set ✗	10	Accuracy OSAS vs. HC (morning): 77%	<0.001
Antonelli Incalzi (2015) [67]	50 C-PAP	41.8 e/h	E-nose (BIONOTE) Pneumopipe + TenaxGR	Internal cross-validation ✓ External validation set ✗		29 consonant change 21 discordant change	
Dragonieri (2015) [61]	19 OS	27.8 e/h	GC-MS (1) E-nose (2) (Cyranose320) Tedlar bags Carboxen and Carbopack cartridges	Internal cross-validation ✓ External validation set ✗	14 ON 20 NO	(1) Accuracy OS vs. ON: 91% (2) AUC OS vs. NO: 1 (2) AUC OS vs. ON:0.7	
Scarlata (2017) [63]	20 hypo 20 non-hypo	13.6 e/h 2.8 e/h	E-nose (BIONOTE) Pneumopipe + TenaxGR	Internal cross-validation ✓ External validation set ✗	56 NO 20 non-hypo COPD 20 ON	Accuracy OSA vs. HC: 0.99 Accuracy OSAS vs. COPD: 0.75	
Benedek (2013) [64]	18	2 e/h	E-nose (Cyranose320) Mylar bags	Internal cross-validation ✗ External validation set ✗	10 habitual snoring	AUROC: 0.84	<0.003
Greulich (2018) [60]	15	26 e/h	Ion mobility mass spectrometry (1) E-nose (Cyranose320) (2)	Internal cross-validation ✓ External validation set ✗	15	(1) AUROC 0.79 (2) AUROC 0.9	0.004 <0.001

Legend: OSAS: obstructive sleep apnea syndrome; AHI: apnea-hypopnea index (e/h: events per hour); AUROC: Area under receiver operating curve; COPD: chronic obstructive pulmonary disease; C-PAP: continuous positive airway pressure; OS: obese OSAS; OVS.: overlap syndrome; ON: obese healthy controls; NO: non-obese healthy controls; hypo: hypoxemic; non-hypo: non hypoxemic; ✓: technical standard satisfied; ✗: technical standard not satisfied.

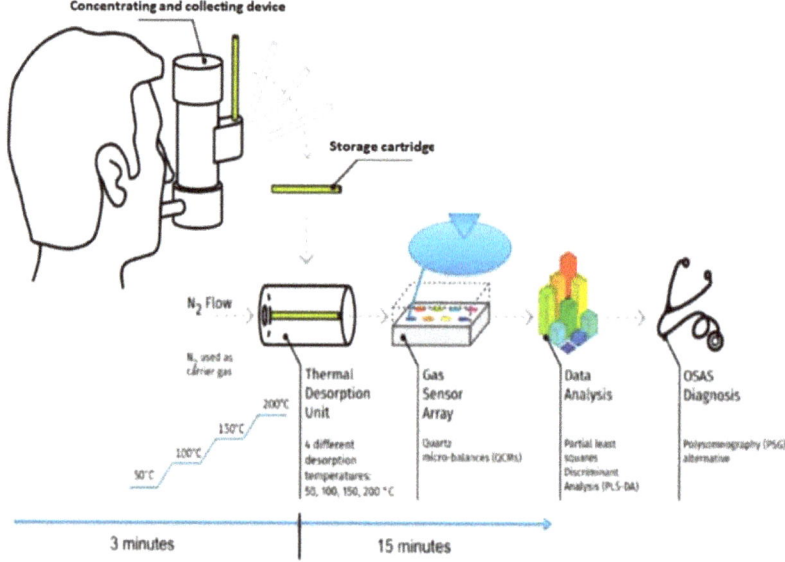

Figure 4. Measure chain of an e-nose based sensor system.

4. Discussion

This updated systematic review confirms the promising role of exhaled breath analysis in the understanding of the mechanisms underpinning disease and its clinical relevance in identifying individuals affected by OSAS. Besides, in addition to previous reviews of the field, it shows that, although the majority of the technical standards proposed by the ERS committee have been followed, more research is needed to stadardize the methodology and hence reduce the variability in the results.

OSAS is characterized by an endothelial dysfunction, arterial stiffening and elevated levels of inflammatory markers as an effect of the intermittent hypoxia caused by the upper airways collapse [71] which increase the risk to develop cardiovascular, metabolic or neurological events. Indeed, hypoxia increases the production of reactive oxygen species (ROS) and thus the oxidative stress, which impairs the phosphorylation of NOS [72,73], reduces the release of nitric oxide and promotes the endothelial dysfunction. Results of studies on FeNO are in line with this notion. Indeed, overall the concentration of FeNO measured at a flow of 50 mL/s is below the 50 ppb, identified by the American Thoracic Society (ATS) as a threshold of the presence of eosinophil airway inflammation. Moreover, the reduced CaNO in the studies of Fortuna and Foresi and its elevation after effective treatment support the existence of an alveolar damage in the disease [23,30]. Furthermore, intermittent hypoxia fosters the development of a chronic inflammation, and this is confirmed by the studies carried out on the EBC. Indeed, pro-inflammatory cytokines increase while anti-inflammatory cytokines decrease in the breath of those patients, and the markers of oxidative stress are elevated in the morning [39,52], as demonstrated also by the studies on the breath pattern [66]. Moreover, inflammatory cells were increased in the muscular layer of patients with OSAS, with CD4+ and activated CD25+ T cells (both increased approximately threefold) predominating. Inflammation was also present in upper airway (UA) mucosa, but with a different pattern consisting of CD8+ (2.8-fold increase) and activated CD25+ (3.2-fold increase) T cell predominance, suggesting that inflammatory cell infiltration affects not only the mucosa, but also the UA muscle of patients with OSAS, this potentially leading to a systemic pro-inflammatory spillover of cytokines and mediators that could promote and amplify chronic inflammatory response [35]. Indeed, these proposed mechanisms are still far from being confirmed and further research is needed to confirm this pathophysiologic mechanism.

Although all the techniques studying volatile and non-volatile compounds are able to discriminate OSAS patients from controls, EBC and the study of volatile organic compounds seem more promising than FeNO for a clinical use. However, efforts are needed to address some the technical and non-technical issues that are hindering the applicability of breath analysis in clinical practice. The role of smoking in increasing inflammation, as well as that of obesity, should be deeper investigated in the studies about OSAS. Besides, issues as the dilution of the EBC [74] or the lack of external validity in most of the studies about volatile organic compounds need to be addressed to increase the reliability of the techniques.

Breathprint analysis of VOCs might have practical applications and could act as a valuable instrument in OSAS management in the next future: considering the high prevalence of OSAS in the general population and its dramatic impact on health status, any effort should be made in order to detect and treat it as soon as possible. Breathprint analysis might complement, or even replace questionnaires in the screening process and, consequently, improve the cost/effectiveness ratio of polysomnography. Furthermore, VOCs analysis could be used to monitor the response to, and the adherence with C-PAP ventilation [57]. Finally, the breath print analysis could help better understanding of the heterogeneity of OSAS phenotypes [69] and define their prognosis, as in other respiratory diseases [75].

5. Conclusions

To conclude, in the era of precision medicine breath analysis, being non-invasiveness, rapid and economic, might play a key role in the understanding of the pathways underpinning OSAS and in the clinical management of the patients affected by the disease.

Author Contributions: P.F., S.S. and R.A.I. participated in the study concept and design. P.F. and S.S. performed the literature search and assessed the eligibility of identified publications independently, R.A.I. and V.C. reviewed the manuscript for important intellectual content. All the authors fulfil authorship criteria, have revised the final version of the manuscript and gave their consent to publication.

Funding: The present study has not received any funding.

Conflicts of Interest: Authors deny any conflict of interest.

References

1. Mehra, R.; Benjamin, E.J.; Shahar, E.; Gottlieb, D.J.; Nawabit, R.; Kirchner, H.L. Association of nocturnal arrhythmias with sleep-disordered breathing: The sleep heart health study. *Am. J. Respir. Crit. Care Med.* **2006**, *173*, 910–916. [CrossRef] [PubMed]
2. Gami, A.S.; Olson, E.J.; Shen, W.K.; Wright, R.S.; Ballman, K.V.; Hodge, D.O.; Herges, R.M.; Howard, D.E.; Somers, V.K. Obstructive Sleep Apnea and the Risk of Sudden Cardiac Death: A Longitudinal Study of 10,701 Adults. *J. Am. Coll. Cardiol.* **2013**, *62*, 610–616. [CrossRef] [PubMed]
3. Peled, N.; Kassirer, M.; Shitrit, D.; Kogan, Y.; Shlomi, D.; Berliner, A.S.; Kramer, M.R. The association of OSA with insulin resistance, inflammation and metabolic syndrome. *Respir. Med.* **2007**, *101*, 1696–1701. [CrossRef] [PubMed]
4. Stone, K.L.; Blackwell, T.L.; Ancoli-Israel, S.; Barrett-Connor, E.; Bauer, D.C.; Cauley, J.A.; Ensrud, K.E.; Hoffman, A.R.; Mehra, R.; Stefanick, M.L.; et al. Sleep Disordered Breathing and Risk of Stroke in Older Community-Dwelling Men. *Sleep* **2016**, *39*, 531–540.
5. Redline, S. Obstructive Sleep Apnea–Hypopnea and Incident Stroke: The Sleep Heart Health Study. *Am. J. Respir. Crit. Care Med.* **2010**, *182*, 1332–1333. [CrossRef]
6. Mulgrew, A.T.; Nasvadi, G.; Butt, A.; Cheema, R.; Fox, N.; Fleetham, J.A.; Ryan, C.F.; Cooper, P.; Ayas, N.T. Risk and severity of motor vehicle crashes in patients with obstructive sleep apnoea/hypopnoea. *Thorax* **2008**, *63*, 536–541. [CrossRef]
7. Schlaud, M.; Urschitz, M.S.; Urschitz-Duprat, P.M.; Poets, C.F.; Urschitz-Duprat, P.M. The German study on sleep-disordered breathing in primary school children: Epidemiological approach, representativeness of study sample, and preliminary screening results. *Paediatr. Périnat. Epidemiol.* **2004**, *18*, 431–440. [CrossRef]

8. Mitchell, R.B.; Kelly, J. Behavior, neurocognition and quality-of-life in children with sleep-disordered breathing. *Int. J. Pediatr. Otorhinolaryngol.* **2006**, *70*, 395–406. [CrossRef]
9. Sabato, R.; Guido, P.; Salerno, F.; Resta, O.; Spanevello, A.; Barbaro, M.F. Airway inflammation in patients affected by obstructive sleep apnea. *Monaldi Arch. Chest Dis.* **2006**, *65*, 102–105. [CrossRef]
10. Holty, J.-E.C.; Owens, D.K.; Dallas, P.; Shekelle, P.; Qaseem, A.; Starkey, M. Management of Obstructive Sleep Apnea in Adults: A Clinical Practice Guideline from the American College of Physicians. *Ann. Intern. Med.* **2013**, *159*, 471–483.
11. Kapur, V.K.; Auckley, D.H.; Chowdhuri, S.; Kuhlmann, D.C.; Mehra, R.; Ramar, K.; Harrod, C.G. Clinical Practice Guideline for Diagnostic Testing for Adult Obstructive Sleep Apnea: An American Academy of Sleep Medicine Clinical Practice Guideline. *J. Clin. Sleep Med.* **2017**, *13*, 479–504. [CrossRef] [PubMed]
12. Scarlata, S.; Pedone, C.; Curcio, G.; Cortese, L.; Chiurco, D.; Fontana, D.; Calabrese, M.; Fusiello, R.; Abbruzzese, G.; Santangelo, S.; et al. Pre-polysomnographic assessment using the Pittsburgh Sleep Quality Index questionnaire is not useful in identifying people at higher risk for obstructive sleep apnea. *J. Med. Screen.* **2013**, *20*, 220–226. [CrossRef] [PubMed]
13. Carpagnano, G.E. Exhaled Breath Analysis and Sleep. *J. Clin. Sleep Med.* **2011**, *7*, S34–S37. [CrossRef] [PubMed]
14. Bikov, A.; Hull, J.H.; Kunos, L.; Information, P.E.K.F.C. Exhaled breath analysis, a simple tool to study the pathophysiology of obstructive sleep apnoea. *Sleep Med. Rev.* **2016**, *27*, 1–8. [CrossRef] [PubMed]
15. Horváth, I.; Barnes, P.J.; Loukides, S.; Sterk, P.J.; Högman, M.; Olin, A.-C.; Amann, A.; Antus, B.; Baraldi, E.; Bikov, A.; et al. A European Respiratory Society technical standard: Exhaled biomarkers in lung disease. *Eur. Respir. J.* **2017**, *49*, 1600965. [CrossRef]
16. Donnelly, L.E.; Barnes, P.J. Expression and Regulation of Inducible Nitric Oxide Synthase from Human Primary Airway Epithelial Cells. *Am. J. Respir. Cell Mol. Boil.* **2002**, *26*, 144–151. [CrossRef] [PubMed]
17. Alving, K.; Weitzberg, E.; Lundberg, J.M. Increased amount of nitric oxide in exhaled air of asthmatics. *Eur. Respir. J.* **1993**, *6*, 1368–1370.
18. Kharitonov, S.; Yates, D.; Robbins, R.; Barnes, P.; Logan-Sinclair, R.; Shinebourne, E. Increased nitric oxide in exhaled air of asthmatic patients. *Lancet* **1994**, *343*, 133–135. [CrossRef]
19. Dweik, R.A.; Boggs, P.B.; Erzurum, S.C.; Irvin, C.G.; Leigh, M.W.; Lundberg, J.O.; Olin, A.-C.; Plummer, A.L.; Taylor, D.R. An Official ATS Clinical Practice Guideline: Interpretation of Exhaled Nitric Oxide Levels (FeNO) for Clinical Applications. *Am. J. Respir. Crit. Care Med.* **2011**, *184*, 602–615. [CrossRef]
20. Zhang, D.; Xiao, Y.; Luo, J.; Wang, X.; Qiao, Y.; Huang, R. Measurement of fractional exhaled nitric oxide and nasal nitric oxide in male patients with obstructive sleep apnea. *Sleep Breath.* **2018**. [CrossRef]
21. Przybyłowski, T.; Bielicki, P.; Kumor, M.; Hildebrand, K.; Maskey-Warzechowska, M.; Fangrat, A.; Górska, K.; Korczyński, P.; Chazan, R. Exhaled nitric oxide in patients with obstructive sleep apnea syndrome. *Pneumonol. Alergol. Polska* **2006**, *74*, 21–25.
22. Petrosyan, M.; Perraki, E.; Simoes, D.; Koutsourelakis, I.; Vagiakis, E.; Roussos, C. Exhaled breath markers in patients with obstructive sleep apnoea. *Sleep Breath.* **2008**, *12*, 207–215. [CrossRef]
23. Fortuna, A.; Miralda, R.; Calaf, N.; Gonzalez, M.; Casan, P.; Mayos, M. Airway and alveolar nitric oxide measurements in obstructive sleep apnea syndrome. *Respir. Med.* **2011**, *105*, 630–636. [CrossRef]
24. Chua, A.-P.; Aboussouan, L.S.; Minai, O.A.; Paschke, K.; Laskowski, D.; Dweik, R.A. Long-Term Continuous Positive Airway Pressure Therapy Normalizes High Exhaled Nitric Oxide Levels in Obstructive Sleep Apnea. *J. Clin. Sleep Med.* **2013**, *9*, 529–535. [CrossRef]
25. Duong-Quy, S.; Hua-Huy, T.; Tran-Mai-Thi, H.-T.; Le-Dong, N.-N.; Craig, T.J.; Dinh-Xuan, A.-T. Study of Exhaled Nitric Oxide in Subjects with Suspected Obstructive Sleep Apnea: A Pilot Study in Vietnam. *Pulm. Med.* **2016**, *2016*, 1–7. [CrossRef]
26. Duarte, R.L.M.; Rabahi, M.F.; Oliveira-E-Sá, T.S.; Magalhães-Da-Silveira, F.J.; Mello, F.C.Q.; Gozal, D. Fractional Exhaled Nitric Oxide Measurements and Screening of Obstructive Sleep Apnea in a Sleep-Laboratory Setting: A Cross-Sectional Study. *Lung* **2019**, *197*, 131–137. [CrossRef]
27. Togores, B.; Agustí, A.G.; Barbé, F. Exhaled Nitric Oxide in Patients with Sleep Apnea. *Sleep* **1999**, *22*, 231–235.
28. Barreto, M.; Montuschi, P.; Evangelisti, M.; Bonafoni, S.; Cecili, M.; Shohreh, R.; Santini, G.; Villa, M.P. Comparison of two exhaled biomarkers in children with and without sleep disordered breathing. *Sleep Med.* **2018**, *45*, 83–88. [CrossRef]

29. Jalil Mirmohammadi, S.; Mehrparvar, A.H.; Safaei, S.; Samimi, E.; Jahromi, M.T. The association between exhaled nitric oxide and sleep apnea: The role of BMI. *Respir. Med.* **2014**, *108*, 1229–1233. [CrossRef]
30. Foresi, A.; Leone, C.; Olivieri, D.; Cremona, G. Alveolar-Derived Exhaled Nitric Oxide Is Reduced in Obstructive Sleep Apnea Syndrome. *Chest* **2007**, *132*, 860–867. [CrossRef]
31. Carpagnano, G.E.; Spanevello, A.; Sabato, R.; DePalo, A.; Turchiarelli, V.; Barbaro, M.P.F. Exhaled pH, exhaled nitric oxide, and induced sputum cellularity in obese patients with obstructive sleep apnea syndrome. *Transl. Res.* **2008**, *151*, 45–50. [CrossRef]
32. Culla, B.; Guida, G.; Brussino, L.; Tribolo, A.; Cicolin, A.; Sciascia, S.; Badiu, I.; Mietta, S.; Bucca, C. Increased oral nitric oxide in obstructive sleep apnoea. *Respir. Med.* **2010**, *104*, 316–320. [CrossRef]
33. DePalo, A.; Carpagnano, G.E.; Spanevello, A.; Sabato, R.; Cagnazzo, M.G.; Gramiccioni, C.; Foschino-Barbaro, M.P. Exhaled NO and iNOS expression in sputum cells of healthy, obese and OSA subjects. *J. Int. Med.* **2008**, *263*, 70–78. [CrossRef]
34. Paulsen, F.P.; Steven, P.; Tsokos, M.; Jungmann, K.; Mueller, A.; Verse, T.; Pirsig, W. Upper Airway Epithelial Structural Changes in Obstructive Sleep-disordered Breathing. *Am. J. Respir. Crit. Care Med.* **2002**, *166*, 501–509. [CrossRef]
35. Boyd, J.H.; Petrof, B.J.; Hamid, Q.; Fraser, R.; Kimoff, R.J. Upper Airway Muscle Inflammation and Denervation Changes in Obstructive Sleep Apnea. *Am. J. Respir. Crit. Care Med.* **2004**, *170*, 541–546. [CrossRef]
36. Paraskakis, E.; Vergadi, E.; Chatzimichael, A.; Bush, A. The Role of Flow-Independent Exhaled Nitric Oxide Parameters in the Assessment of Airway Diseases. *Curr. Top. Med. Chem.* **2016**, *16*, 1631–1642. [CrossRef]
37. Hua-Huy, T.; Le-Dong, N.-N.; Duong-Quy, S.; Luchon, L.; Rouhani, S.; Dinh-Xuan, A.T. Increased alveolar nitric oxide concentration is related to nocturnal oxygen desaturation in obstructive sleep apnoea. *Nitric Oxide* **2015**, *45*, 27–34. [CrossRef]
38. Ip, M.S.M.; Lam, B.; Chan, L.-Y.; Zheng, L.; Tsang, K.W.T.; Fung, P.C.W.; Lam, W.-K. Circulating Nitric Oxide Is Suppressed in Obstructive Sleep Apnea and Is Reversed by Nasal Continuous Positive Airway Pressure. *Am. J. Respir. Crit. Care Med.* **2000**, *162*, 2166–2171. [CrossRef]
39. Olopade, C.O.; Christon, J.A.; Zakkar, M.; Swedler, W.I.; Rubinstein, I.; Hua, C.-W.; Scheff, P.A. Exhaled Pentane and Nitric Oxide Levels in Patients with Obstructive Sleep Apnea. *Chest* **1997**, *111*, 1500–1504. [CrossRef]
40. Liu, J.; Li, Z.; Liu, Z.; Zhu, F.; Li, W.; Jiang, H. Exhaled nitric oxide from the central airway and alveoli in OSAHS patients: The potential correlations and clinical implications. *Sleep Breath.* **2016**, *20*, 145–154. [CrossRef] [PubMed]
41. Gut, G.; Tauman, R.; Greenfeld, M.; Armoni-Domany, K.; Sivan, Y. Nasal nitric oxide in sleep-disordered breathing in children. *Sleep Breath.* **2016**, *20*, 303–308. [CrossRef] [PubMed]
42. Kis, A.; Meszaros, M.; Tarnoki, D.L.; Tarnoki, A.D.; Lazar, Z.; Horvath, P.; Kunos, L.; Bikov, A. Exhaled carbon monoxide levels in obstructive sleep apnoea. *J. Breath Res.* **2019**. [CrossRef] [PubMed]
43. Greulich, T.; Hattesohl, A.; Grabisch, A.; Koepke, J.; Schmid, S.; Noeske, S. Detection of obstructive sleep apnoea by an electronic nose. *Eur. Respir. J.* **2013**, *42*, 145–155. [CrossRef] [PubMed]
44. Paget-Brown, A.O.; Ngamtrakulpanit, L.; Smith, A.; Bunyan, D.; Hom, S.; Nguyen, A.; Hunt, J.F. Normative Data for pH of Exhaled Breath Condensate. *Chest* **2006**, *129*, 426–430. [CrossRef] [PubMed]
45. Lloberes, P.; Sánchez-Vidaurre, S.; Ferré, Á.; Cruz, M.J.; Lorente, J.; Sampol, G.; Morell, F.; Muñoz, X. Effect of Continuous Positive Airway Pressure and Upper Airway Surgery on Exhaled Breath Condensate and Serum Biomarkers in Patients with Sleep Apnea. *Arch. Bronconeumol.* **2014**, *50*, 422–428. [CrossRef]
46. Antonopoulou, S.; Loukides, S.; Papatheodorou, G.; Roussos, C.; Alchanatis, M. Airway inflammation in obstructive sleep apnea: Is leptin the missing link? *Respir. Med.* **2008**, *102*, 1399–1405. [CrossRef]
47. Carpagnano, G.E.; Kharitonov, S.A.; Resta, O.; Foschino-Barbaro, M.P.; Gramiccioni, E.; Barnes, P.J. Increased 8-Isoprostane and Interleukin-6 in Breath Condensate of Obstructive Sleep Apnea Patients. *Chest* **2002**, *122*, 1162–1167. [CrossRef] [PubMed]
48. Li, Y.; Chongsuvivatwong, V.; Geater, A.; Liu, A. Exhaled breath condensate cytokine level as a diagnostic tool for obstructive sleep apnea syndrome. *Sleep Med.* **2009**, *10*, 95–103. [CrossRef]
49. Carpagnano, G.E.; Spanevello, A.; Sabato, R.; DePalo, A.; Palladino, G.P.; Bergantino, L.; Barbaro, M.P.F. Systemic and airway inflammation in sleep apnea and obesity: The role of ICAM-1 and IL-8. *Transl. Res.* **2010**, *155*, 35–43. [CrossRef]

50. Karamanlı, H.; Özol, D.; Ugur, K.S.; Yıldırım, Z.; Armutçu, F.; Bozkurt, B. Influence of CPAP treatment on airway and systemic inflammation in OSAS patients. *Sleep Breath.* **2014**, *18*, 251–256. [CrossRef]
51. Li, Y.; Chongsuvivatwong, V.; Geater, A.; Liu, A. Are Biomarker Levels a Good Follow-Up Tool for Evaluating Obstructive Sleep Apnea Syndrome Treatments? *Respir. Int. Rev. Thorac. Dis.* **2008**, *76*, 317–323. [CrossRef]
52. Carpagnano, G.E.; Kharitonov, S.A.; Resta, O.; Foschino-Barbaro, M.P.; Gramiccioni, E.; Barnes, P.J. 8-Isoprostane, a Marker of Oxidative Stress, Is Increased in Exhaled Breath Condensate of Patients With Obstructive Sleep Apnea After Night and Is Reduced by Continuous Positive Airway Pressure Therapy. *Chest* **2003**, *124*, 1386–1392. [CrossRef]
53. Fernandez Alvarez, R.; Rubinos Cuadrado, G.; Alonso Arias, R.; Cascon Hernandez, J.A.; Palomo Antequera, B.; Iscar Urrutia, M. Snoring as a Determinant Factor of Oxidative Stress in the Airway of Patients with Obstructive Sleep Apnea. *Lung* **2016**, *194*, 469–473. [CrossRef]
54. Malakasioti, G.; Alexopoulos, E.; Befani, C.; Tanou, K.; Varlami, V.; Ziogas, D. Oxidative stress and inflammatory markers in the exhaled breath condensate of children with OSA. *Sleep Breath.* **2012**, *16*, 703–708. [CrossRef]
55. Vlasic, V.; Trifunovic, J.; Cepelak, I.; Nimac, P.; Topic, R.Z.; Dodig, S. Urates in exhaled breath condensate of children with obstructive sleep apnea. *Biochem. Med.* **2011**, *21*, 139–144. [CrossRef]
56. Goldbart, A.D.; Krishna, J.; Li, R.C.; Serpero, L.D.; Gozal, D. Inflammatory Mediators in Exhaled Breath Condensate of Children with Obstructive Sleep Apnea Syndrome. *Chest* **2006**, *130*, 143–148. [CrossRef]
57. Carpagnano, G.E.; Resta, O.; De Pergola, G.; Sabato, R.; Barbaro, M.P.F. The role of obstructive sleep apnea syndrome and obesity in determining leptin in the exhaled breath condensate. *J. Breath Res.* **2010**, *4*, 36003. [CrossRef]
58. Schulz, S.; Dickschat, J.S. Bacterial volatiles: The smell of small organisms. *Nat. Prod. Rep.* **2007**, *24*, 814–842. [CrossRef]
59. Finamore, P.; Scarlata, S.; Incalzi, R.A. Breath analysis in respiratory diseases: State-of-the-art and future perspectives. *Expert Rev. Mol. Diagn.* **2019**, *19*, 47–61. [CrossRef]
60. Greulich, T.; Fischer, H.; Lubbe, D.; Nell, C.; Baumbach, J.I.; Koehler, U.; Boeselt, T.; Vogelmeier, C.; Koczulla, A.R. Obstructive sleep apnea patients can be identified by ion mobility spectrometry-derived smell prints of different biological materials. *J. Breath Res.* **2018**, *12*, 026006. [CrossRef]
61. Dragonieri, S.; Porcelli, F.; Longobardi, F.; Carratu, P.; Aliani, M.; Ventura, V.A.; Tutino, M.; Quaranta, V.N.; Resta, O.; De Gennaro, G. An electronic nose in the discrimination of obese patients with and without obstructive sleep apnoea. *J. Breath Res.* **2015**, *9*, 26005. [CrossRef]
62. Aoki, T.; Nagaoka, T.; Kobayashi, N.; Kurahashi, M.; Tsuji, C.; Takiguchi, H. Editor's highlight: Prospective analyses of volatile organic compounds in obstructive sleep apnea patients. *Toxicol. Sci. Off. J. Soc. Toxicol.* **2017**, *156*, 362–374. [CrossRef]
63. Scarlata, S.; Pennazza, G.; Santonico, M.; Santangelo, S.; Bartoli, I.R.; Rivera, C.; Vernile, C.; De Vincentis, A.; Incalzi, R.A. Screening of Obstructive Sleep Apnea Syndrome by Electronic-Nose Analysis of Volatile Organic Compounds. *Sci. Rep.* **2017**, *7*, 11938. [CrossRef] [PubMed]
64. Benedek, P.; Lazar, Z.; Bikov, A.; Kunos, L.; Katona, G.; Horváth, I. Exhaled biomarker pattern is altered in children with obstructive sleep apnoea syndrome. *Int. J. Pediatr. Otorhinolaryngol.* **2013**, *77*, 1244–1247. [CrossRef]
65. Dragonieri, S.; Quaranta, V.N.; Carratu, P.; Ranieri, T.; Resta, O. Exhaled breath profiling in patients with COPD and OSA overlap syndrome: A pilot study. *J. Breath Res.* **2016**, *10*, 41001. [CrossRef]
66. Kunos, L.; Bikov, A.; Lazar, Z.; Korosi, B.Z.; Benedek, P.; Losonczy, G. Evening and morning exhaled volatile compound patterns are different in obstructive sleep apnoea assessed with electronic nose. *Sleep Breath.* **2015**, *19*, 247–253. [CrossRef]
67. Antonelli Incalzi, R.; Pennazza, G.; Scarlata, S.; Santonico, M.; Vernile, C.; Cortese, L. Comorbidity modulates non invasive ventilation-induced changes in breath print of obstructive sleep apnea syndrome patients. *Sleep Breath.* **2015**, *19*, 623–630. [CrossRef]
68. Schwarz, E.I.; Martinez-Lozano Sinues, P.; Bregy, L.; Gaisl, T.; Garcia Gomez, D.; Gaugg, M.T. Effects of CPAP therapy withdrawal on exhaled breath pattern in obstructive sleep apnoea. *Thorax* **2016**, *71*, 110–117. [CrossRef]
69. Scarlata, S.; Pennazza, G.; Santonico, M.; Pedone, C.; Incalzi, R.A. Exhaled breath analysis by electronic nose in respiratory diseases. *Expert Rev. Mol. Diagn.* **2015**, *15*, 1–24. [CrossRef]

70. Pennazza, G.; Santonico, M.; Scarlata, S.; Santangelo, S.; Grasso, S.; Zompanti, A.; Incalzi, R.A. A Non Invasive Sensor System for the Screening of Obstructive Sleep Apnea Syndrome. *Proceedings* **2017**, *1*, 426. [CrossRef]
71. Wang, J.; Yu, W.; Gao, M.; Zhang, F.; Gu, C.; Yu, Y.; Wei, Y. Impact of Obstructive Sleep Apnea Syndrome on Endothelial Function, Arterial Stiffening, and Serum Inflammatory Markers: An Updated Meta-analysis and Metaregression of 18 Studies. *J. Am. Hear. Assoc.* **2015**, *4*, e002454. [CrossRef] [PubMed]
72. Thomas, S.R.; Chen, K.; Keaney, J.F. Hydrogen peroxide activates endothelial nitric-oxide synthase through coordinated phosphorylation and dephosphorylation via a phosphoinositide 3-kinase-dependent signaling pathway. *J. Biol. Chem.* **2002**, *277*, 6017–6024. [CrossRef] [PubMed]
73. Tanaka, T.; Nakamura, H.; Yodoi, J.; Bloom, E.T. Redox regulation of the signaling pathways leading to eNOS phosphorylation. *Free Radic. Biol. Med.* **2005**, *38*, 1231–1242. [CrossRef] [PubMed]
74. Bikov, A.; Gálffy, G.; Tamasi, L.; Lazar, Z.; Losonczy, G.; Horváth, I. Exhaled breath condensate pH is influenced by respiratory droplet dilution. *J. Breath Res.* **2012**, *6*, 46002. [CrossRef]
75. Finamore, P.; Pedone, C.; Scarlata, S.; Di Paolo, A.; Grasso, S.; Santonico, M.; Pennazza, G.; Antonelli Incalzi, R. Validation of exhaled volatile organic compounds analysis using e-nose as index of COPD severity. *Int. J. Chron. Obstruct. Pulmon. Dis.* **2018**, *13*, 1441–1448. [CrossRef]

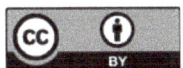

© 2019 by the authors. Licensee MDPI, Basel, Switzerland. This article is an open access article distributed under the terms and conditions of the Creative Commons Attribution (CC BY) license (http://creativecommons.org/licenses/by/4.0/).

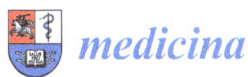

Brief Report

Risk Assessment for Self Reported Obstructive Sleep Apnea and Excessive Daytime Sleepiness in a Greek Nursing Staff Population

Alexia Alexandropoulou [1], Georgios D. Vavougios [2], Chrissi Hatzoglou [1,3], Konstantinos I. Gourgoulianis [3] and Sotirios G. Zarogiannis [1,3,*]

1. Department of Physiology, Faculty of Medicine, University of Thessaly, BIOPOLIS, 41500 Larissa, Greece
2. Department of Neurology, Athens Naval Hospital, 11521 Athens, Greece
3. Department of Respiratory Medicine, Faculty of Medicine, University of Thessaly, BIOPOLIS, 41500 Larissa, Greece
* Correspondence: szarog@med.uth.gr; Tel.: +30-2410-685558

Received: 15 June 2019; Accepted: 5 August 2019; Published: 12 August 2019

Abstract: *Background and objectives*: The risk assessment of Obstructive Sleep Apnea (OSA) and Excessive Daytime Sleepiness (EDS) in specific occupational populations is important due to its association with morbidity. The aim of the present study was to identify the risk of OSA development and EDS in a Greek nursing staff population. *Materials and Methods*: In this cross-sectional study a total of 444 nurses, 56 males (age = 42.91 ± 5.76 years/BMI = 27.17 ± 4.32) and 388 females (age = 41.41 ± 5.92 years/BMI = 25.08 ± 4.43) working in a Greek secondary and tertiary hospital participated during the period from 18 January 2015 to 10 February 2015. The participants completed the Berlin Questionnaire (BQ), concerning the risk for OSA and the Epworth Sleepiness Scale (ESS), concerning the EDS. The work and lifestyle habits of the participants were correlated with the results of the questionnaires. *Results*: According to the BQ results 20.5% (n = 91) of the nursing staff was at high risk for OSA. Increased daytime sleepiness affected 27.7% (n = 123) of the nurses according to ESS results. Nurses at risk for Obstructive Sleep Apnea Syndrome (OSAS), positive for both BQ and ESS, were 7.66% (n = 34). Out of the nurses that participated 77% (n = 342) were working in shifts status and had significant meal instability (breakfast p < 0.0001, lunch p < 0.0001, dinner p = 0.0008). *Conclusions*: The population at high risk for OSA and EDS in the nursing staff was found to be 20% and 28% respectively. High risk for OSAS was detected in 7.66% of the participants. The high risk for OSA and EDS was the same irrespective of working in shift status. In specific, nursing population age was an independent predictor for high risk for OSA and skipping lunch an independent predictor of daytime sleepiness.

Keywords: Berlin Questionnaire; Epworth Sleepiness Scale; nursing staff; Obstructive Sleep Apnea Syndrome; risk assessment

1. Introduction

The World Health Organization (WHO) indicates that Obstructive Sleep Apnea Syndrome (OSAS) is a preventable lung disease [1]. Most patients with this syndrome exhibit no detectable respiratory dysfunction when awake while OSAS appears in all age groups. However, in the adult population the incidence of this syndrome increases with age and is clearly linked with excessive daytime sleepiness (EDS) [1–3].

The prevalence of this syndrome is probably higher than the one presumed due to underdiagnosis. Thus, OSAS constitutes an important public health issue [4–7]. It is estimated that 26% of the worldwide adult population is at high risk for developing the syndrome [4]. Epidemiological studies indicate that the exact determination of OSAS prevalence is difficult due to different methodological approaches [3,8,9]. Studies from USA, Australia, India, China and Korea report that the prevalence in the general adult population spans from 3 to 7% in men and 2 to 5% in women to more than 49% depending on age and gender [5–7,9–15]. This reported non-uniformity of the prevalence in 4 different continents strengthens the notion that the disease is common but the prevalence in the community needs to be studied more rigorously in order to avoid underdiagnosis [4,8].

The investigation of OSAS in the context of specific occupations is of high interest given that its occurrence may be associated with working conditions that do not only induce the disease but also affect the job performance and overall health [16–18]. A study on American and Canadian police officers showed that this specific population has at least one sleep disorder. Moreover, one third of the study population, suffered from OSAS (33.6%) [19]. Another study in young male Korean soldiers using the Berlin Questionnaire (BQ) reported a prevalence of 8.1% of OSA [20]. In a similar study conducted in the staff of an Iranian hospital again with the BQ tool, it was found that 6.9% were at high risk for OSAS. Finally, a study in 21 nurses, showed that according to the BQ, 24% were at high risk for OSA, but subsequent polysomnography revealed that 43% of them were diagnosed with OSAS [16].

No studies exist in the Greek population regarding the risk assessment of self-reported OSA and EDS in specific occupational groups. Given that the nursing staff work several times in shift status, which has been implicated in the induction of OSAS [21,22], we hypothesized that this population would be under risk for developing OSA and EDS, due to their sleep fragmentation. Thus, the aim of the present study was to identify the nursing population at high risk for OSA and EDS in a secondary and tertiary hospital in Greece.

2. Materials and Methods

2.1. Study Population

The study population consisted of 444 nurses working in the University Hospital and the General Hospital of Larissa during the period 18 January 2015 to 10 February 2015 who volunteered to participate in the study. In total, 530 questionnaires were distributed by the primary author in personal communication with the potential participants. The potential participants were given a week to complete the questionnaires and were asked to put them in an un-named envelope and hand them to a designated administrative officer of each hospital sector (Medical, Surgical and Intensive Care) for collection by the primary author. Out of the 530 questionnaires 449 were returned to the primary author. Out of the 449 questionnaires, 5 were not fully completed and were thus excluded from the study, leading to a final number of 444 questionnaires included in the study. The study involved 56 male (12.6%) and 388 female (87.4%) nurses, regardless of educational level and work experience, from all nursing departments. All participants provided demographic information such as gender, age, height, weight, smoking habits, skipping meals and whether they worked under night shifts. The Ethics Committee of the University Hospital of Larissa approved the research protocol (Protocol number: 1/14-1-2015).

2.2. OSAS and EDS Assessment Tools

In order to assess the risk of OSAS the Greek version of the Berlin Questionnaire (BQ) was used [23]. The BQ contains 10 questions that are divided in 3 categories. In the first category the questions aim at identifying the self-reported snoring behavior along with witnessed apneas during sleep by the partner. The second category assesses self-reported fatigue after sleep and the third assesses the presence of obesity or history of hypertension. If two of the categories of the BQ are positive, then the participant is assigned as being at high risk for OSAS.

In order to assess the excessive daytime sleepiness, the Greek version of the Epworth Sleepiness Scale (ESS) was used [24]. ESS aims at the quantification of daytime sleepiness though a set of self-reported incidents of dozing in eight different setting during the day and the scoring spans from 0 to 24. A participant in high risk for daytime sleepiness has a score of 10 or higher.

2.3. Statistical Analysis

Statistical analysis was performed by EpiInfo v. 7.0 (CDC, Atlanta, GA, USA), the SPSS 24.0 Software (IBM Corporation, New York, NY, USA) and GraphPad Prism v. 8.1 (San Diego, CA, USA). Fisher's exact was used to assess differences among proportions. The Mann Whitney test was used to assess differences between two groups. Multivariate logistic regression was performed as in other similar studies [25]. The Forward Conditional Logistic Regression Model was used to perform multivariate analyses of the effect of univariate predictors on the likelihood of belonging to the high OSA probability (based on BQ) or high daytime sleepiness (Based on Epworth Scale) groups, while controlling for potential confounders. Values are expressed as mean ± S.D. A p value of less than 0.05 was deemed significant.

3. Results

3.1. Study Population

Out of the 530 questionnaires that were distributed, 444 were completed and collected, providing a responsiveness rate of 83.8%. The demographics of the study population along with lifestyle habits are shown in Table 1.

Table 1. Characteristics of the participants in the study.

	Males	Females	p Value
Gender (%)	56 (12.6%)	388 (87.4%)	-
Age (years)	42.91 ± 5.76	41.41 ± 5.92	0.047
Height (m)	1.78 ± 0.06	1.65 ± 0.05	<0.001
Weight (kg)	86.05 ± 14.30	67.91 ± 12.03	<0.001
BMI	27.17 ± 4.32	25.08 ± 4.43	<0.001
Smokers—Yes(#)	29 (51.79%)	171 (44.07%)	0.39
Pack Years (#)	14.61 ± 11.31	15.78 ± 11.18	0.59
Alcohol Consumption—Yes (%)	40 (70.42%)	192 (49.48%)	0.004
Working on Night Shifts—Yes (%)	44 (78.57%)	287 (73.97%)	0.52
Night Shifts per month (#)	4.43 ± 1.87	6.25 ± 2.25	<0.001

3.2. BQ and ESS Questionnaire Results

The results of the BQ questionnaire showed that 20% (n = 91) of the participants were found to be at high risk for OSAS as opposed to 80% (353) that were found to be at low risk for OSAS (Figure 1A). With regards to the ESS questionnaire 28% (n = 123) of the participants were found to be at high risk for EDS as opposed to the 72% (n = 321) that were found at low risk (Figure 1B).

More importantly a fraction of these two groups mounting to 8% (n = 34) were found to be at concomitant high risk for both OSA and EDS, thus at OSAS risk.

There were no differences in the proportions of male and female nurses that were positive in BQ (p > 0.99) or ESS (p = 0.75). Working under night shift status did not result in a higher proportion of nurses to test positive in BQ (p = 0.69), but resulted in a higher proportion of nurses testing positive in ESS (p = 0.005).

Another significant finding of our study was that the nursing staff working on shift work status reported skipping meals significantly more than the nurses not under shift status that had a greater stability in maintaining the three main meals of the day as shown in Figure 2.

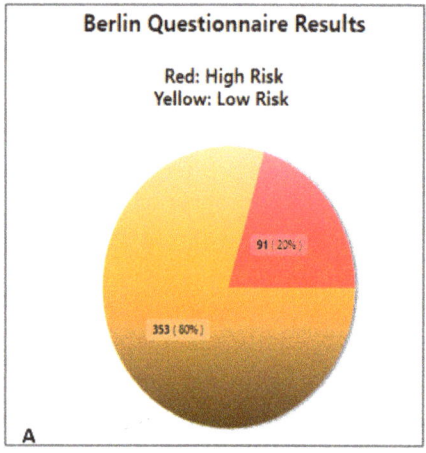
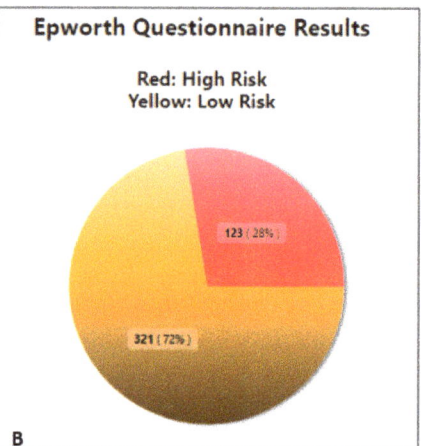

Figure 1. (**A**) Results of the Berlin Questionnaire (BQ) showing 20% of the participants at high risk for Obstructive Sleep Apnea (OSA). (**B**) Results of the Epworth Sleepiness Scale (ESS) showing 28% of the participants at high risk for Excessive Daytime Sleepiness (EDS).

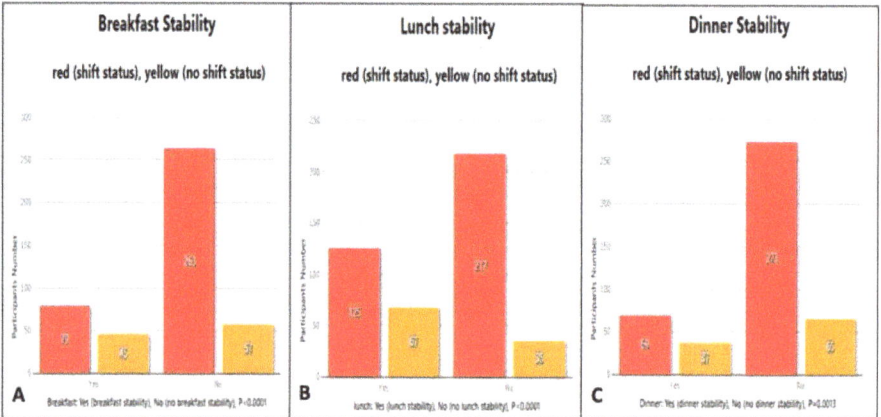

Figure 2. Significant meal instability (skipping of a meal) in the nursing staff working on shift work status regarding (**A**) breakfast, (**B**) lunch and (**C**) dinner.

The Forward Conditional Binary Logistic Regression model was subsequently used in order to determine the effects of age, sex, alcohol consumption, education level, smoking status and breakfast/lunch/dinner skipping on the likelihood of belonging to the (a) high OSA risk and (b) high daytime sleepiness groups. Age was the single independent predictor of belonging to the high risk OSA group [OR: 0.959 (95% CI: 0.922–0.998), p-value = 0.038], whereas lunch skipping [OR: 1.631, (95% CI: 1.060–2.509), p = 0.026] independently predicted higher daytime sleepiness.

4. Discussion

The aim of the present investigation was the identification of the risk for OSA and EDS in the nursing population of a secondary and tertiary hospital in Greece using the standard questionnaires. Our results showed that the nursing population at high risk for OSA was 20%, while that of EDS was 28%. The fraction of the study population that was at high risk for both, and therefore at high OSAS risk, was 8%. Moreover, according to our results, working in shift status did not directly affect the risk for OSA. However, it significantly worsened EDS in the nursing population. It has to be taken into account that the sensitivity and specificity of BQ for OSA diagnosis in the Greek population has been shown to be 76% and 40%, respectively, while the Greek version of ESS had also proved a useful tool for the identification of EDS in Greece [23,24]. In the studied population after multivariate logistic regression it was shown that age was a significant predictor of high risk for OSA, while skipping lunch was an independent prognosticator for high EDS risk. Aging is a known risk factor for OSA development so our result is in line with the literature [26]. As far as lunch skipping is concerned, a study that focused on the daytime sleepiness of subjects during the Ramadan intermittent fasting showed that this intentional prolonged daytime abstinence from food intake, induced an increase in the objective and subjective daytime sleepiness of the subjects [27]. Thus, based on the ESS scores of the participants of our study, we are in agreement with the notion that daytime food abstinence increases the propensity for subjective daytime sleepiness.

There is lack of studies on the risk assessment for OSA and EDS in nursing populations in Greece, so our results cannot be compared to the published literature. However, a similar study performed in the USA in nurses working in shift status using the BQ, showed that 24% of participants were at risk for OSA [16]. Although our study had a sample size nearly 20-fold bigger the above-mentioned results are comparable to ours that showed that 20% of the population was at high risk for OSA. On the other hand, in the study of Geiger-Brown et al., after polysomnography 43% of the participating nurses were diagnosed with sleep-disordered breathing, therefore if we extrapolate these findings to our study, we should expect a significantly higher number of nurses with OSAS in our sample. This was a limitation of our study but is the topic of a new investigation currently underway. A previous Greek study has shown that in subjects that underwent polysomnography, OSAS was diagnosed five times more in men than women, nevertheless using the BQ we did not detect such a difference between genders [28].

Data stemming from other occupational groups have reported comparable results. A cross-sectional and prospective cohort study in police officers in North America that involved a 10-fold greater population ($n = 4957$) than ours indicated that 40.1% of the police staff had at least one sleep disorder [29]. The most important of these disorders that was observed in 33.6% was OSAS. A total of 28.5% of the police staff also had EDS and the significant possibility to sleep during driving (once a month).

The failure of sleep replenishment during the day and the abnormality of melatonin levels affects the daily fatigue and reduces the quality of life [18]. In our study, 28% of the nurses were found to have EDS according to the ESS results. This finding is alerting under the rationale that sleep deprivation can lead to reduced concentration and productivity, and also in increased traffic and occupational accidents and injuries, as well as chronic diseases (cardiovascular and metabolic) and reduced quality of life [16–18,21,22]. Although no relevant data exists in the literature regarding Greece in order to be able to compare our findings, we are in good agreement with studies performed in nurses in New Zealand (that reported 33.75% of positive ESS) and Sweden (that reported 32.5% of positive ESS with a cut-off of 9 that was different from the one in our study that was 10) [30,31]. Our results were higher than a recent study performed in China that reported 16.1% positive ESS but the cut-off the authors used was 14, therefore these results are not directly comparable with the current study [32]. Another important finding of our study was that the nursing population working in shift status had significant instability in all three main meals of the day as determined by the self-report of participants of meal skipping. It has been reported that the instability of meals induces increases in body weight and thus BMI [18]. Obesity is a known risk factor for OSAS and furthermore a specific type of sleep apnea is observed in this population, the Obesity Hypoventilation Syndrome (OHS) [3,16]. Indeed, in our study the participants that were found to be in the high risk for OSA based on BQ results were significantly heavier that the ones in the low-risk group. Moreover, shift status has been implicated in the induction of OSAS [21,22]. Shift-work disrupts the expression of circadian genes and sleep patterns, deregulates metabolic processes and can cause sleep apnea and several disorders linked to OSAS like cardiovascular disorders and obesity [33].

There were some limitations in the current study. The population of our study was young since most nurses were in their early forties predominantly. Additionally, our sample comprised predominantly of females and this may have diluted the significance of our results. Finally, all participants were originating from a single geographic area and thus further multicenter studies are needed.

5. Conclusions

In conclusion, we found that the risk for OSA and EDS in a nursing population of a secondary and tertiary hospital in Greece was 20% and 28% respectively. At high risk for OSAS were 8% of the participants (positive BQ and ESS simultaneously). Moreover, we found that nurses that work under night shift status had significant meal instability, which is a risk factor of obesity, which is in turn linked to OSAS development. However, we detected no differences in OSAS risk between these two groups of the population assessed. Further study of the population under high risk for OSAS of this study involving polysomnography assessment is needed.

Author Contributions: Conceptualization, S.G.Z.; data curation, A.A. and S.G.Z.; formal analysis, A.A.; investigation, A.A.; methodology, G.D.V., C.H., K.I.G. and S.G.Z.; project administration, S.G.Z.; resources, C.H., K.I.G. and S.G.Z.; supervision, S.G.Z.; visualization, A.A. and S.G.Z.; writing—original draft preparation, A.A. and S.G.Z.; writing—review and editing, A.A., G.D.V., C.H., K.I.G. and S.G.Z.

Funding: This research received no external funding.

Conflicts of Interest: The authors declare no conflict of interest.

References

1. Veale, D. Chronic respiratory care and rehabilitation in France. *Chron. Respir. Dis.* **2006**, *3*, 215–216. [CrossRef] [PubMed]
2. Berry, R.B.; Budhiraja, R.; Gottlieb, D.J.; Gozal, D.; Iber, C.; Kapur, V.K.; Marcus, C.L.; Mehra, R.; Parthasarathy, S.; Quan, S.F.; et al. Rules for scoring respiratory events in sleep: Update of the 2007 AASM manual for the scoring of sleep and associated events. *J. Clin. Sleep Med.* **2012**, *8*, 597–619. [CrossRef] [PubMed]
3. Jennum, P.; Riha, R.L. Epidemiology of sleep apnoea/hypopnoea syndrome and sleep-disordered breathing. *Eur. Respir. J.* **2009**, *33*, 907–914. [CrossRef] [PubMed]
4. Carlucci, M.; Smith, M.; Corbridge, S.J. Poor sleep, hazardous breathing: an overview of obstructive sleep apnea. *Nurse Pract.* **2013**, *38*, 20–28. [CrossRef] [PubMed]
5. Peppard, P.E.; Young, T.; Barnet, J.H.; Palta, M.; Hagen, E.W.; Hla, K.M. Increased prevalence of sleep-disordered breathing in adults. *Am. J. Epidemiol.* **2013**, *177*, 1006–1014. [CrossRef] [PubMed]
6. Heinzer, R.; Vat, S.; Marques-Vidal, P.; Marti-Soler, H.; Andries, D.; Tobback, N.; Mooser, V.; Preisig, M.; Malhotra, A.; Waeber, G.; et al. Prevalence of sleep-disordered breathing in the general population: The HypnoLaus study. *Lancet Respir. Med.* **2015**, *3*, 310–318. [CrossRef]
7. Simpson, L.; Hillman, D.R.; Cooper, M.N.; Ward, K.L.; Hunter, M.; Cullen, S.; James, A.; Palmer, L.J.; Mukherjee, S.; Eastwood, P. High prevalence of undiagnosed obstructive sleep apnoea in the general population and methods for screening for representative controls. *Sleep Breath.* **2013**, *17*, 967–973. [CrossRef] [PubMed]
8. Punjabi, N.M. The epidemiology of adult obstructive sleep apnea. *Proc. Am. Thorac. Soc.* **2008**, *5*, 136–143. [CrossRef]
9. Mirrakhimov, A.E.; Sooronbaev, T.; Mirrakhimov, E.M. Prevalence of obstructive sleep apnea in Asian adults: a systematic review of the literature. *BMC Pulm. Med.* **2013**, *13*, 10. [CrossRef]
10. Sharma, S.K.; Ahluwalia, G. Epidemiology of adult obstructive sleep apnoea syndrome in India. *Indian J. Med. Res.* **2010**, *131*, 171–175.
11. Mahboub, B.; Afzal, S.; Alhariri, H.; Alzaabi, A.; Vats, M.; Soans, A. Prevalence of symptoms and risk of sleep apnea in Dubai, UAE. *Int. J. Gen. Med.* **2013**, *6*, 109–114. [PubMed]

12. BaHammam, A.S.; Alrajeh, M.S.; Al-Jahdali, H.H.; BinSaeed, A.A. Prevalence of symptoms and risk of sleep apnea in middle-aged Saudi males in primary care. *Saudi Med. J.* **2008**, *29*, 423–426. [PubMed]
13. Kang, K.; Seo, J.G.; Seo, S.H.; Park, K.S.; Lee, H.W. Prevalence and related factors for high-risk of obstructive sleep apnea in a large Korean population: Results of a questionnaire-based study. *J. Clin. Neurol.* **2014**, *10*, 42–49. [CrossRef] [PubMed]
14. Tufik, S.; Santos-Silva, R.; Taddei, J.A.; Bittencourt, L.R.A. Obstructive Sleep Apnea Syndrome in the Sao Paulo Epidemiologic Sleep Study. *Sleep Med.* **2010**, *11*, 441–446. [CrossRef] [PubMed]
15. Akkoyunlu, M.E.; Altin, R.; Kart, L.; Atalay, F.; Örnek, T.; Bayram, M.; Tor, M. Investigation of obstructive sleep apnoea syndrome prevalence among long-distance drivers from Zonguldak, Turkey. *Multidiscip. Respir. Med.* **2013**, *8*, 2–7. [CrossRef]
16. Geiger-Brown, J.; Rogers, V.E.; Han, K.; Trinkoff, A.; Bausell, R.B.; Scharf, S.M. Occupational screening for sleep disorders in 12-h shift nurses using the Berlin Questionnaire. *Sleep Breath.* **2013**, *17*, 381–388. [CrossRef] [PubMed]
17. Simpson, G. Circadian rhythm sleep disorders. *J. R. Coll. Physicians Edinb.* **2011**, *41*, 94.
18. Rajaratnam, S.M.W.; Howard, M.E.; Grunstein, R.R. Sleep loss and circadian disruption in shift work: health burden and management. *Med. J. Aust.* **2013**, *199*, 11–15. [CrossRef]
19. Ko, H.S.; Kim, M.Y.; Kim, Y.H.; Lee, J.; Park, Y.G.; Moon, H.B.; Kil, K.C.; Lee, G.; Kim, S.J.; Shin, J.C. Obstructive sleep apnea screening and perinatal outcomes in Korean pregnant women. *Arch. Gynecol. Obstet.* **2013**, *287*, 429–433. [CrossRef]
20. Lee, Y.C.; Eun, Y.G.; Shin, S.Y.; Kim, S.W. Prevalence of snoring and high risk of obstructive sleep apnea syndrome in young male soldiers in Korea. *J. Korean Med. Sci.* **2013**, *28*, 1373–1377. [CrossRef]
21. Laudencka, A.; Klawe, J.J.; Tafil-Klawe, M.; Zlomanczuk, P. Does night-shift work induce apnea events in osbtructive sleep apnea patients? *J. Physiol. Pharmacol.* **2007**, *58*, 345–347.
22. Paciorek, M.; Korczynski, P.; Bielicki, P.; Byśkiniewicz, K.; Zieliński, J.; Chazan, R. Obstructive sleep apnea in shift workers. *Sleep Med.* **2011**, *12*, 274–277. [CrossRef]
23. Bouloukaki, I.; Komninos, I.D.; Mermigkis, C.; Micheli, K.; Komninou, M.; Moniaki, V.; Mauroudi, E.; Siafakas, N.M.; Schiza, S.E. Translation and validation of Berlin questionnaire in primary health care in Greece. *BMC Pulm. Med.* **2013**, *13*, 6. [CrossRef]
24. Tsara, V.; Serasli, E.; Amfilochiou, A.; Constantinidis, T.; Christaki, P. Greek version of the Epworth Sleepiness Scale. *Sleep Breath.* **2004**, *8*, 91–95. [CrossRef]
25. Romandini, M.; Gioco, G.; Perfetti, G.; Deli, G.; Staderini, E.; Laforì, A. The association between periodontitis and sleep duration. *J. Clin. Periodontol.* **2017**, *44*, 490–501. [CrossRef]
26. Gaspar, L.S.; Alvaro, A.R.; Moita, J.; Cavadas, C. Obstructive sleep apnea and hallmarks of aging. *Trends Mol. Med.* **2017**, *23*, 675–692. [CrossRef]
27. Roky, R.; Chapotot, F.; Benchekroun, M.T.; Benaji, B.; Hakkou, F.; Elkhalifi, H.; Buguet, A. Daytime sleepiness during Ramadan intermittent fasting: polysomnographic and quantitative waking EEG study. *J. Sleep Res.* **2003**, *12*, 95–101. [CrossRef]
28. Vagiakis, E.; Kapsimalis, F.; Lagogianni, I.; Perraki, H.; Minaritzoglou, A.; Alexandropoulou, K.; Roussos, C.; Kryger, M. Gender differences on polysomnographic findings in Greek subjects with obstructive sleep apnea syndrome. *Sleep Med.* **2006**, *7*, 424–430. [CrossRef]
29. Barger, L.K.; Lockley, S.W.; Shea, S.A.; Wang, W.; Landrigan, C.P.; O'Brien, C.S.; Qadri, S.; Sullivan, J.P.; Cade, B.E.; Epstein, L.J.; et al. Sleep disorders, health and safety in Police Officers. *Jama* **2013**, *306*, 2567–2578.
30. Gander, P.; OKeeffe, K.; Santos-Fernandez, E.; Annette, H.; Leonie, W.; Jinny, W. Fatigue and nurses' work patterns: An online questionnaire survey. *Int. J. Nurs. Stud.* **2019**, *98*, 67–74. [CrossRef]
31. Brown, J.G.; Wieroney, M.; Blair, L.; Zhu, S.; Warren, J.; Scharf, S.M.; Hinds, P.S. Measuring subjective sleepiness at work in hospital nurses: Validation of a modified delivery format of the Karolinska Sleepiness Scale. *Sleep Breath.* **2014**, *18*, 731–739. [CrossRef]

32. Chen, L.; Luo, C.; Liu, S.; Chen, W.; Liu, Y.; Li, Y.; Du, Y.; Zou, H.; Pan, J. Excessive daytime sleepiness in general hospital nurses: prevalence, correlates, and its association with adverse events. *Sleep Breath.* **2019**, *23*, 209–216. [CrossRef]
33. Khan, S.; Duan, P.; Yao, L.; Hou, H. Shiftwork-mediated disruptions of circadian rhythms and sleep homeostasis cause serious health problems. *Int. J. Genomics* **2018**, *2018*, 8576890. [CrossRef]

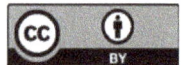

© 2019 by the authors. Licensee MDPI, Basel, Switzerland. This article is an open access article distributed under the terms and conditions of the Creative Commons Attribution (CC BY) license (http://creativecommons.org/licenses/by/4.0/).

MDPI
St. Alban-Anlage 66
4052 Basel
Switzerland
Tel. +41 61 683 77 34
Fax +41 61 302 89 18
www.mdpi.com

Medicina Editorial Office
E-mail: medicina@mdpi.com
www.mdpi.com/journal/medicina

www.ingramcontent.com/pod-product-compliance
Lightning Source LLC
LaVergne TN
LVHW070542100526
838202LV00012B/358